SAUNDERS
ELSEVIER

©2007, Elsevier Limited. All rights reserved.

No part of this publication may be reproduced, stored in a retrieval system, or transmitted in any form or by any means, electronic, mechanical, photocopying, recording or otherwise, without the prior permission of the Publishers. Permissions may be sought directly from Elsevier's Health Sciences Rights Department, 1600 John F. Kennedy Boulevard, Suite 1800, Philadelphia, PA 19103-2899, USA: phone: (+1) 215 239 3804; fax: (+1) 215 239 3805; or, e-mail: healthpermissions@elsevier.com. You may also complete your request on-line via the Elsevier homepage (http://www.elsevier.com), by selecting 'Support and contact' and then 'Copyright and Permission'.

First published 2007

ISBN-13: 978-0-7020-2818-2
ISBN: 10: 0 7020 2818 5

British Library Cataloguing in Publication Data
A catalogue record for this book is available from the British Library

Library of Congress Cataloging in Publication Data
A catalog record for this book is available from the Library of Congress

Knowledge and best practice in this field are constantly changing. As new research and experience broaden our knowledge, changes in practice, treatment and drug therapy may become necessary or appropriate. Readers are advised to check the most current information provided (i) on procedures featured or (ii) by the manufacturer of each product to be administered, to verify the recommended dose or formula, the method and duration of administration, and contraindications. It is the responsibility of the practitioner, relying on their own experience and knowledge of the patient, to make diagnoses, to determine dosages and the best treatment for each individual patient, and to take all appropriate safety precautions. To the fullest extent of the law, neither the publisher nor the author assumes any liability for any injury and/or damage.

The Publisher

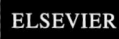 your source for books, journals and multimedia in the health sciences

www.elsevierhealth.com

Working together to grow
libraries in developing countries

www.elsevier.com | www.bookaid.org | www.sabre.org

ELSEVIER   BOOK AID International   Sabre Foundation

The Publisher

The publisher's policy is to use **paper manufactured from sustainable forests**

Printed in China

Handbook of Equine Respiratory Endoscopy

Safia Barakzai BVSc MSc DipECVS Cert Equine Surgery (Soft Tissue) MRCVS

Department of Veterinary Clinical Studies
Royal (Dick) School of Veterinary Studies
University of Edinburgh
UK

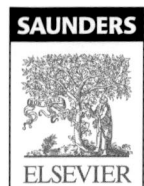

Edinburgh London New York Oxford Philadelphia St Louis Sydney Toronto 2007

For Elsevier:

Commissioning Editor: Joyce Rodenhuis
Development Editor: Rita Demetriou-Swanwick
Project Manager: David Fleming
Designer: Andy Chapman
Illustrations Manager: Bruce Hogarth
Illustrator: Sam Elhurst

Handbook of Equine Respiratory Endoscopy

Contents

Dedication vi

Foreword vii

Acknowledgments viii

Chapter 1 Endoscopic equipment 3

Chapter 2 Practical guide to equine respiratory endoscopy ... 11

Chapter 3 Nasal cavities 15

Chapter 4 Pharynx 31

Chapter 5 Guttural pouches 49

Chapter 6 Larynx 67

Chapter 7 Trachea and bronchi 89

Chapter 8 High-speed treadmill endoscopy 105

Chapter 9 Sinoscopy 119

Index 133

To my mother and father, Lorna and Zaman, for their unfailing support and encouragement

Foreword

The use of endoscopy in veterinary practice has become commonplace over the last decade, such that almost every practice dealing with horses now owns a fibreoptic or videoendoscope. The equine upper and lower respiratory tract suffers a huge array of disorders and therefore not surprisingly, the vast majority of endoscopy in equine clinical practice concerns examination of the respiratory tract. This handbook concentrates on the more common abnormalities found in the respiratory system.

This handbook aims to educate general equine practitioners and veterinary students to become familiar with the normal endoscopic appearance and normal variations of the equine upper and lower respiratory tract, and from there, to recognise and interpret abnormalities of these areas. The highly visual nature of the book allows the reader to compare what they see endoscopically in their own cases with the disorders illustrated in this text and it would be a useful book for the practitioner to keep in the car as a quick reference and for client education.

A concise outline of aetiology, diagnosis, treatment and prognosis is given for each disorder, thus giving key information which can help the practitioner make a diagnosis and also provide information that can be easily relayed to the client. This handbook is not aimed to provide exhaustive information on all disorders of the equine respiratory tract, and further reading lists are provided at the end of each chapter which will enable the reader to research individual disorders in more detail. This book will make a valuable addition to all equine practitioners' collections.

Professor Paddy Dixon
University of Edinburgh

Acknowledgments

I wish to thank and acknowledge all the equine clinicians at the Royal (Dick) School of Veterinary Studies, Edinburgh who were involved in the many cases photographed for this handbook.

I am particularly grateful to Professor Paddy Dixon for provision of many images for this manuscript, and for his advice and instruction over the years.

Thanks also to Justin Perkins, John Keen, Dr Hester McAllister, Thomas Leaman and Dr Eric Strand for providing images, and to Dr Jim Schumacher and Dr Derek Knottenbelt for their editorial guidance.

Chapter preview

Selecting an endoscope for equine respiratory endoscopy 3
Length and diameter of endoscope 3
Fiberoptic vs. videoendoscopes 3
Light sources 5

Maintenance of endoscopes 5
Cleaning and disinfection 5
Sterilization 5
Testing 6
Storage 6

Accessories 6
Biopsy and grasping forceps 6
Simple and guarded aspiration/delivery catheters 7
Lance catheters 7

Further reading 8

1: Endoscopic equipment

Selecting an endoscope for equine respiratory endoscopy

Length and diameter of endoscope

A wide variety of endoscopes are available for examination of the equine respiratory tract. For general equine practice, an endoscope should have a wide range of applications in order to make it both a useful diagnostic instrument and a sound economic investment.

The external diameter of the endoscope is important; an endoscope with a small diameter (7–9 mm) will allow examination of the nasal meatuses, the guttural pouches and the airways of foals or small ponies. An endoscope of sufficient length to reach the 'sump' of the trachea for collection of respiratory secretions in adult horses (approximately 100–110 cm) is ideal. Longer endoscopes (>160 cm) are required for bronchoscopy or for collection of broncho-alveolar lavage fluid from adult horses. Equine gastroscopy requires an endoscope with a 250–300 cm working length.

Fiberoptic (Fig. 1-1) vs. videoendoscopes (Fig. 1-2)

These two systems differ in the way that images are collected and transmitted to the eyepiece or monitor. Fiberoptic images are transmitted from the subject, through long thin fibers of optical glass, into a magnifying eyepiece. The optical fibers are quite sensitive to damage which may be caused by excessive bending or general wear and tear, and broken fibers are represented by black dots on the image. Using a 'coupler', an external video camera can be attached to the eyepiece of a fiberoptic endoscope to enable transmission of the image to a monitor screen. However, the quality of image is not as good as that seen directly through the eyepiece. The main advantage of fiberoptic endoscope systems is that they are easily portable and inexpensive, and therefore, they are often chosen by clinicians who work in ambulatory practice.

Videoendoscopes provide a higher quality image than do fiberoptic endoscopes but are more expensive. Videoendoscopes produce an image at the objective lens at the distal tip of the insertion tube (the portion of the scope that is inserted into the patient) (Fig. 1-3) which is sensed by a charged couple device (CCD) chip. This image is transmitted electronically via wires along the length of the endoscope to a processor, which converts the signal back into a standard video signal. This video signal can then be displayed on a

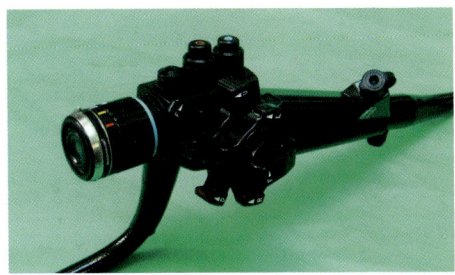

Fig. 1-1: Fiberoptic scope with eyepiece.

Handbook of Equine Respiratory Endoscopy

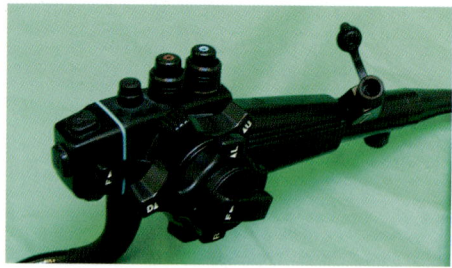

Fig. 1-2: Videoendoscope.

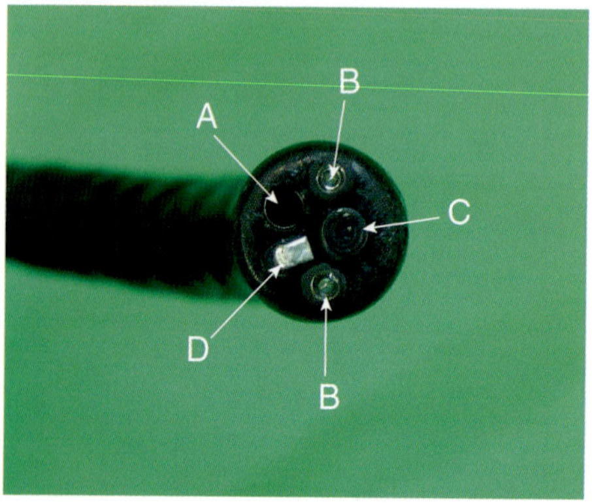

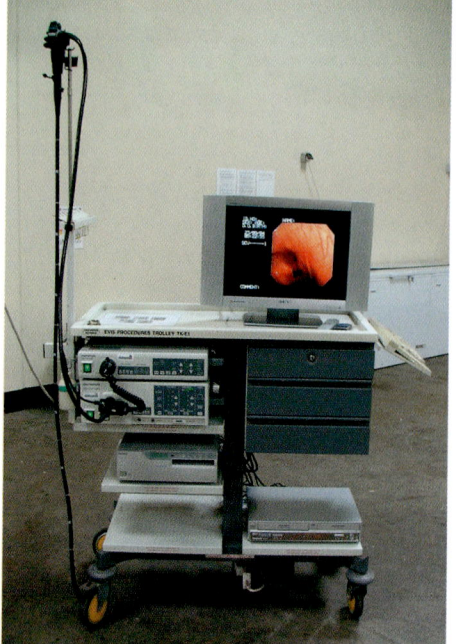

Fig. 1-3: Tip of the insertion tube of a videoendoscope:
A = instrument channel,
B = light guide bundles,
C = CCD bundle,
D = air/water feed channel.

Fig. 1-4: Videoendoscope set-up: the endoscope uses a halogen light source and output from the endoscope is connected to a monitor, printer and DVD/video recorder.

Chapter 1: **Endoscopic equipment**

monitor and recorded on a videotape or DVD, or printed (Fig. 1-4). Videoendoscopes are often connected to large monitors and recording devices, and therefore most systems are not readily portable. They should be considered an essential addition to any equine practice with a clinic facility. Smaller, more portable videoendoscope units with built-in digital recording systems are now becoming available for use in equine practice.

Light sources

Halogen 'cold' light sources are the most commonly used for equine respiratory endoscopy and are available as compact and light units (Fig. 1-5). A light source with an integral air feed/pump allows the tip of the endoscope to be flushed with water and air to clear it of debris. Xenon light sources produce a higher-intensity, cleaner light than do halogen light sources, but are considerably more expensive to buy and maintain.

Maintenance of endoscopes

Cleaning and disinfection

The endoscope should be cleaned thoroughly after every endoscopic examination to minimize cross-contamination of pathogenic microbes between horses. After endoscopically examining a horse with potentially infectious respiratory disease (e.g. strangles or influenza), the endoscope should be fully sterilized.

Manufacturers of endoscopes provide cleaning instructions in their manufacturer's manual that should be strictly adhered to. Both the external surface of the endoscope and the air/water and biopsy channels should be cleaned and flushed after every procedure; first with an enzymatic cleaning solution, then with water, and finally with air to dry the channels. Some endoscopes are fully submersible, but the eyepiece end of older fiberoptic endoscopes may not be waterproof and immersion in water can result in serious damage. When the endoscope has been used, a channel cleaning brush should be inserted in all the channels at least once daily. Cleaning brushes come in various sizes and in reusable and disposable versions.

Sterilization

Flexible endoscopes can be sterilized by immersion in 2% gluteraldehyde solution for several hours (see guidelines provided by manufacturers of the endoscope and the disinfectant),

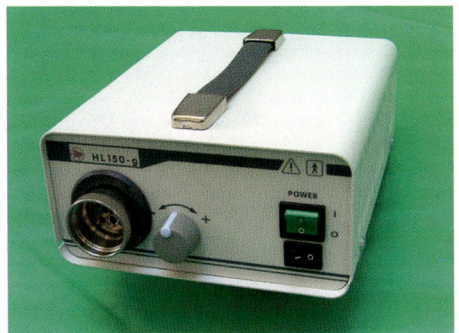

Fig. 1-5: Small halogen light source with air feed, suitable for use with a fiberoptic endoscope.

5

followed by thorough rinsing of the exterior and all the channels in sterile water, because gluteraldehyde is very irritant to tissues. Full sterilization is not routinely carried out after every use because repeated sterilization may predispose to leakages. Ethylene oxide sterilization is a good alternative to wet sterilization, but the ethylene oxide sterilization procedure may take up to 72 hours, rendering the endoscope out of use for this time.

Testing

All endoscopes should be tested regularly for leakages in the channels using the manufacturer's leakage testing equipment. This enables small leaks to be identified before irreparable damage occurs. Regular maintenance programs are also essential to ensure that the optical systems, the sheath and the channels are in good working order.

Storage

Endoscopes, and particularly fiberoptic endoscopes, should be stored in a hanging position with the insertion tube straight. This prevents damage to optical fibers, stops liquid from settling in the channels and prevents the insertion tube from becoming deformed. They should not be stored coiled inside their cases.

Accessories

Biopsy and grasping forceps

A variety of biopsy and grasping forceps are available for endoscopic use. For general practice, the most useful all-round instrument is either standard or serrated fenestrated cup biopsy forceps (Fig. 1-6a, b). These forceps have a rounded, atraumatic end, which, when shut, can be also be used to facilitate endoscopy of the guttural pouches (see Chapter 5). 'Basket' forceps (Fig. 1-6b) can be useful for retrieving larger masses, such as chondroids or foreign bodies from the respiratory tract.

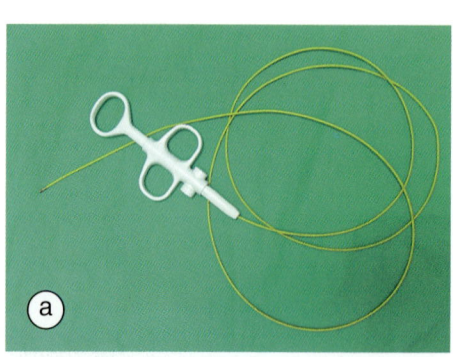 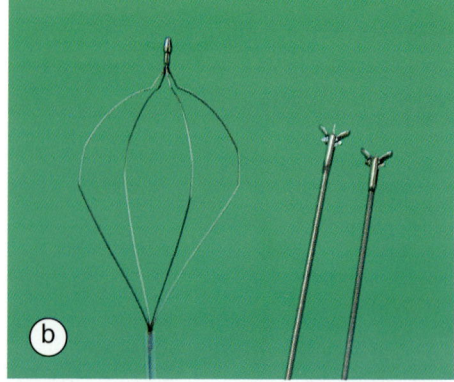

Fig. 1-6: Transendoscopic biopsy and grasping forceps.
a) Whole instrument with plastic handle to open/close jaws.
b) Close-up of jaws. Left to right: basket grasping forceps, standard fenestrated cup biopsy forceps with needle and standard fenestrated cup biopsy forceps.

Chapter 1: **Endoscopic equipment**

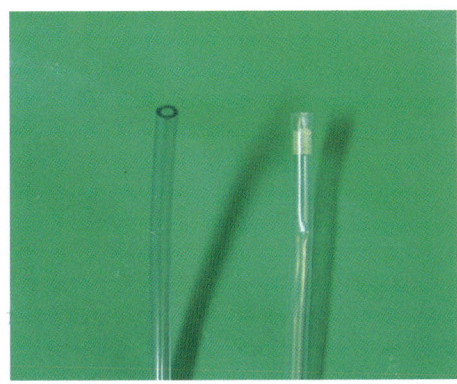

Fig. 1-7: Simple aspiration catheter (left) and aspiration catheter with glycol plug tip (right) (Mila International endoscopic delivery catheter).

Simple and guarded aspiration/delivery catheters (Fig. 1-7)

Simple aspiration/delivery catheters are commonly used for delivery of fluid or medication and aspiration of samples (e.g. tracheal washes) for cytological examination. One end has a 'female' luer lock to which a syringe can be attached. Simple Teflon™, polypropylene, polyethylene or polyurethane catheters are available in lengths of up to 240 cm and external diameters of 1.8 mm or 2.4 mm. Some companies manufacture aspiration catheters that contain a glycol plug in the tip, which reduces contamination of the catheter's lumen by microbes as the catheter is advanced through the biopsy channel of the endoscope. This glycol plug is pushed out of the catheter after the endoscope is positioned in the required area and allows an uncontaminated sample to be collected for bacteriological culture.

'Double-guarded' aspiration catheters are also available (e.g. Mila International endoscopic microbiological aspiration catheter). These catheters contain a glycol plug in the outer catheter which is pushed out after the endoscope is in place, allowing extrusion of an inner catheter which is used to retrieve an uncontaminated sample.

Lance catheters (Fig. 1-8)

These are catheters with needles attached to one end, designed for aspiration and injection of fluids. They are useful for a variety of endoscopic applications, including injecting ethmoidal hematomas with formalin, injecting sites with local anesthetic prior to surgery

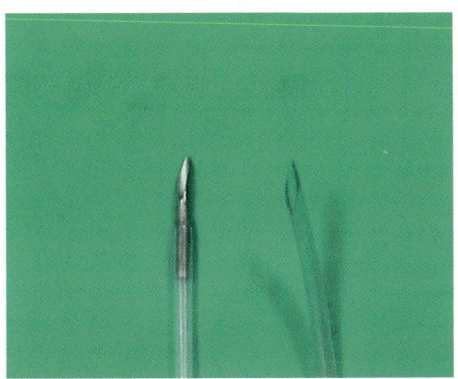

Fig. 1-8: Lance catheters: Mila International 'Lance-a-lot' (left) and homemade lance catheter (right) made by cutting a plain Teflon™ catheter obliquely with a scalpel blade – this type of catheter is sharp enough to penetrate soft masses such as ethmoidal hematomas, but not more dense tissues.

(e.g. for biopsy of masses and laser surgery of the upper respiratory tract), and taking fine-needle aspirates from lesions. If the tissue to be injected/aspirated is quite soft (e.g. an ethmoidal hematoma), a simple aspiration/delivery catheter, cut obliquely with a scalpel blade to a form a sharp point, may provide an inexpensive alternative. Lance catheters made in this way are safe to pass unguarded through the biopsy channel of the endoscope, because they are not sharp enough to damage the inner sleeve. Homemade lance catheters can also be constructed by fixing a short hypodermic needle into the end of an aspiration catheter that has been passed through the biopsy channel of the endoscope. However, there is a risk that the needle may become detached from the tubing when it is inside the horse or inside the biopsy channel of the endoscope, causing significant damage.

FURTHER READING

Lamar AM 1996 Standard fiberoptic and video endoscopic equipment. In: Equine Endoscopy 2nd edn. JL Traub-Dargatz, CM Brown eds. Mosby, St. Louis, pp 13–27

Chapter preview

Normal anatomy 15

Tips for endoscopic examination   18

Abnormalities 18

    Extraluminal narrowing of the nasal cavities 18

    Nasal mycosis 20

    Rhinitis sicca 20

    Nasal polyps 20

    Neoplasia of the nasal cavities 22

    Apical infection of the rostral maxillary cheek teeth 23

    Progressive ethmoidal hematomas 24

    Discharges from, or abnormalities of, the sinus drainage angle 24

    Foreign bodies 24

    Nasal septum deviation 27

    Choanal atresia 27

Further reading 29

but is not an accurate predictor of the presence of dynamic URT disorders which occur only during exercise, and is certainly no substitute for high-speed treadmill endoscopy (see Chapter 8).

Some veterinarians perform endoscopy in the standing horse immediately after exercise in the hope of diagnosing dynamic URT disorders. However, most dynamic causes of URT obstruction resolve within seconds after the cessation of fast work. Additionally, subtleties in laryngeal asymmetry/asynchrony, which can be observed in the quiet, resting horse, may be more difficult to assess immediately post exercise.

FURTHER READING

Ducharme NG, Hackett RP, Fubini SL, et al. 1991 The reliability of endoscopic examination in assessment of laryngeal function in horses. Part II: Side of examination, influence of re-examination and sedation. Veterinary Surgery 20:180–184

Guidelines for endoscopic examination for the purpose of laryngeal evaluation. 2003. In: Proceedings of the Havemeyer Foundation Workshop on Idiopathic Laryngeal Hemiplegia, P Dixon, E Robinson, JF Wade eds. R & W Publications, Newmarket, p 95

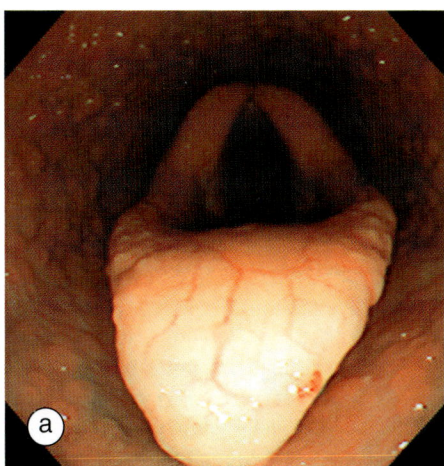 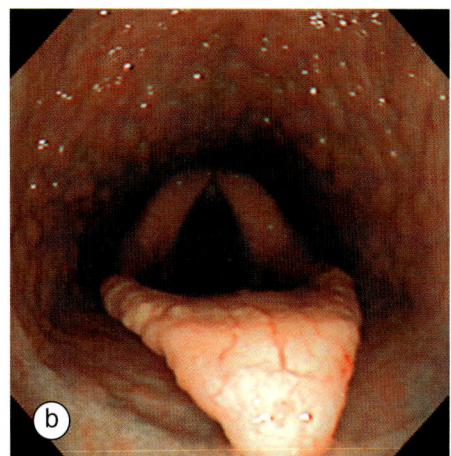

Fig. 2-2: Perspective artifacts arise from the obliquity due to viewing the pharynx/larynx via one nostril.
a) View of the larynx with the endoscope passed up the right nostril.
b) View of the same larynx with the endoscope passed up the left nostril.

When performing bronchoscopy or broncho-alveolar lavage, sedation using a combination of an alpha-2 agonist (e.g. xylazine, romifidine or detomodine) and butorphanol will facilitate passage of the endoscope into the bronchi and reduces the coughing reflex. Spraying local anesthetic solution, such as lidocaine, into the bronchioles may facilitate bronchoscopy, but is not usually required for performing transendoscopic broncho-alveolar lavage.

Epistaxis is an uncommon complication of upper respiratory endoscopy. It usually occurs if the endoscope is inadvertently inserted into the middle or common meatus (instead of the ventral meatus) and advanced blindly. This can result in trauma to the very vascular mucosa of the nasal chonchae or the ethmoturbinates, which are situated at the caudal aspect of the middle meatus. The risk of epistaxis can be minimized by careful initial placement of the endoscope in the ventral meatus and continuous visualization of the position of the endoscope tip as it is inserted. The hemorrhage resulting from mucosal trauma can appear quite substantial (particularly to the horse's owner) but in the absence of clotting dyscrasias is seldom clinically significant.

Timing of endoscopic examination

The vast majority of respiratory endoscopy is performed with the horse standing at rest, and this is adequate unless exercise-related causes of upper airway obstruction (such as intermittent dorsal displacement of the soft palate, vocal fold or arytenoid cartilage collapse, nasopharyngeal collapse and axial deviation of the aryepiglottic folds) are suspected. To assess laryngeal function and to grade horses with recurrent laryngeal neuropathy, arytenoid abduction should be evaluated after swallowing (which can be induced by flushing water through the biopsy channel of the endoscope), and during bilateral nasal occlusion. Nasal occlusion simulates the increased negative pressures generated in the URT during exercise,

2: Practical guide to equine respiratory endoscopy

Specific tips for endoscopic examination of different regions of the equine upper respiratory tract (URT), and for performing endoscopically guided procedures are discussed in more detail in the relevant chapters.

Restraint of the horse

Most horses require some form of restraint before endoscopy of the respiratory tract can be performed safely and efficiently. If nasopharyngeal or laryngeal functions are to be evaluated, chemical sedation should not be used because it significantly affects the appearance and movement of these structures. Typical artefacts seen in sedated horses are rostral displacement of the palatopharyngeal arch (Fig. 6-15) and a reduction in symmetry or synchrony of movement of the arytenoid cartilages. Application of a nose twitch often provides sufficient restraint to allow passage of the endoscope into the respiratory tract to the level of the carina. For a fractious, unsedated horse, endoscopy may be easier to perform with the horse twitched and restrained in stocks (Fig. 2-1). Occasionally, chemical restraint is required in order to ensure the safety of both the horse and attending personnel.

Perspective artefacts arise due to the obliquity caused by viewing the pharynx/larynx via one nasal cavity (Fig. 2-2). Therefore, if the same nostril is used as a matter of course (the author routinely uses the right nostril), the endoscopist learns to recognize and compensate for this obliquity. Varying the nostril through which the endoscope is introduced has been shown to decrease the repeatability of laryngeal grading. If there is any doubt as to the significance of apparent asymmetry of a structure/structures, the procedure should be repeated with the endoscope inserted into the contralateral nasal cavity.

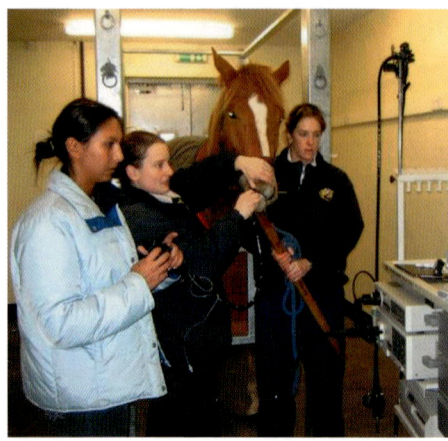

Fig. 2-1: Performing an endoscopic examination at rest – most horses can be endoscoped using a nose twitch as restraint. This does not have a significant effect on arytenoid cartilage movement. Note that the endoscope is routinely passed up the right nasal cavity, and the horse is restrained with a twitch from the other side.

11

Chapter preview

Restraint of the horse 11

Timing of endoscopic examination 12

Further reading 13

3: Nasal cavities

Normal anatomy (Figs 3-1 and 3-2)

The left and right nasal cavities extend from the external nares rostrally to their communication with the nasopharynx (choanae) caudally. The false nostril is situated on the dorso-lateral aspect of the nostril, therefore to avoid inserting the endoscope into this blind-ending sac, it should always be introduced ventrally, at the more axial aspect of either nostril.

The left and right nasal cavities are completely separated by a cartilaginous nasal septum, which slots into the vomer bone at its ventral aspect. Each nasal cavity is divided into four communicating compartments (meatuses) by the largely cartilaginous dorsal and ventral nasal conchae. The dorsal meatus is 'n'-shaped and is situated dorsal to the dorsal concha (Fig. 3-3). The middle meatus is located between the dorsal and ventral concha, and whilst the medial aspect of the middle meatus (which communicates with the common meatus) can be visualized endoscopically, the lateral portion of the middle meatus is usually too narrow to pass an endoscope into (Figs. 3-2, 3-4). The common meatus is positioned between the conchae and the nasal septum and is continuous with the other meatuses. Together, the common and middle meatuses make a 'y'-shape which can be visualized endoscopically (Fig. 3-4). The ventral meatus is 'u'-shaped and is located ventral to the ventral concha (Fig. 3-5). The nasal conchae and nasal septum are covered with vascular respiratory mucosa, in which superficial blood vessels may be identified easily in the normal horse.

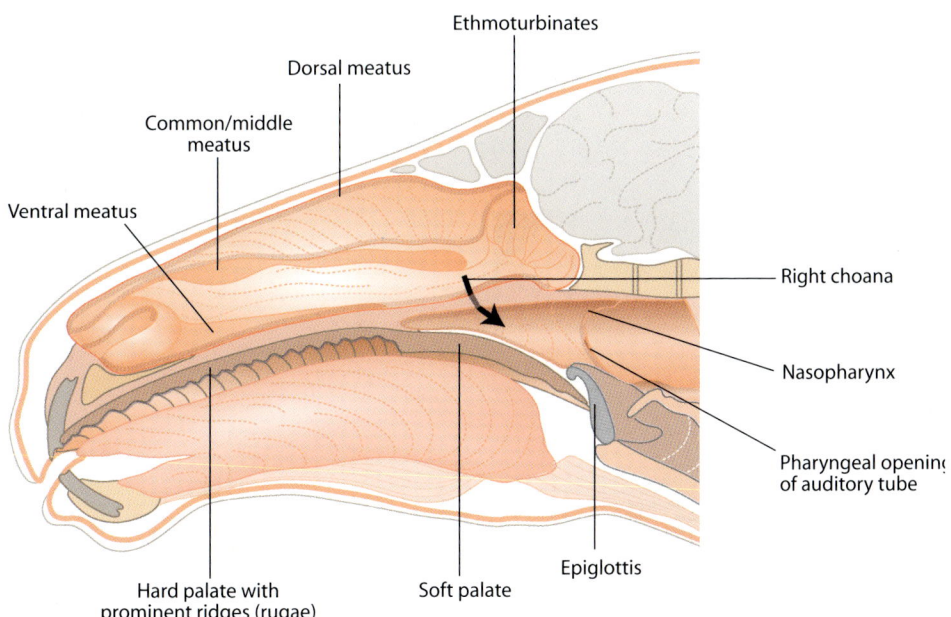

Fig. 3-1: Median section of equine head with the nasal septum removed.

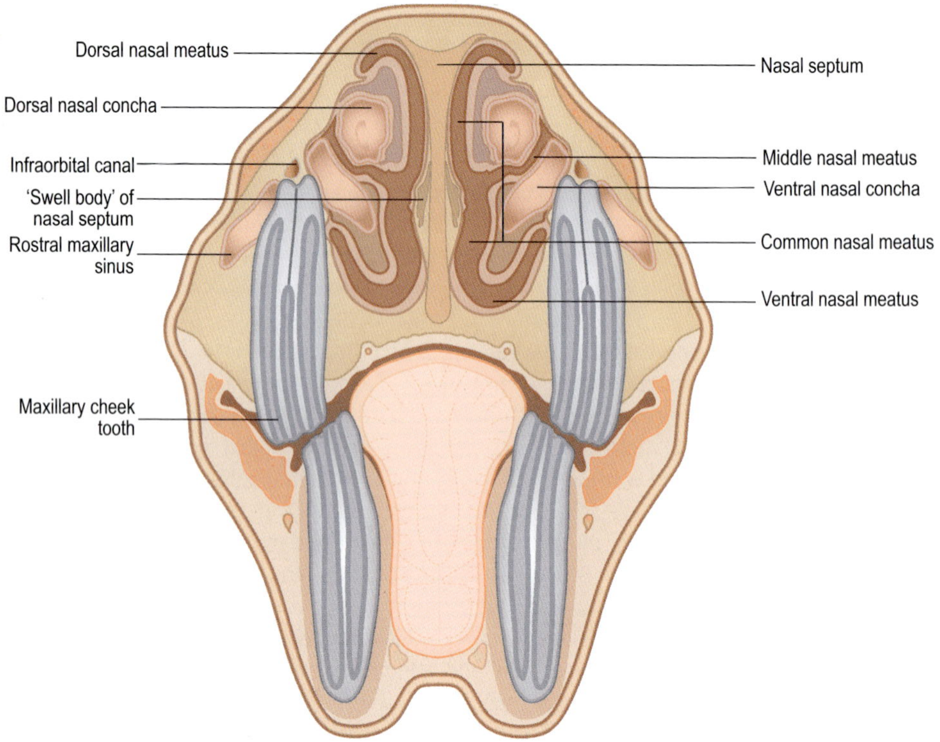

Fig. 3-2: Transverse section through equine skull at the level of the rostral maxillary sinus.

Labels: Dorsal nasal meatus; Dorsal nasal concha; Infraorbital canal; 'Swell body' of nasal septum; Rostral maxillary sinus; Maxillary cheek tooth; Nasal septum; Middle nasal meatus; Ventral nasal concha; Common nasal meatus; Ventral nasal meatus.

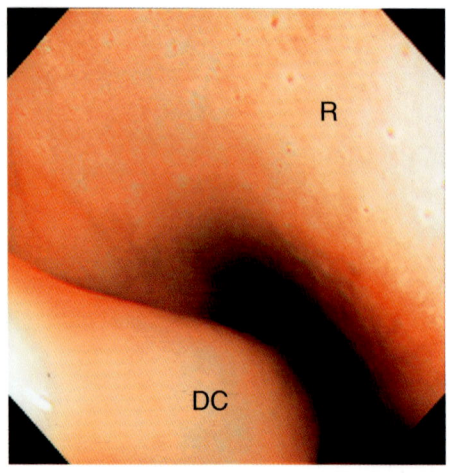

Fig. 3-3: Dorsal nasal meatus of the right nasal cavity in the normal horse – note the 'n'-shape of this meatus, bordered ventrally by the dorsal concha (DC), and dorsally by the roof of the nasal cavity (R).

Chapter 3: **Nasal cavities**

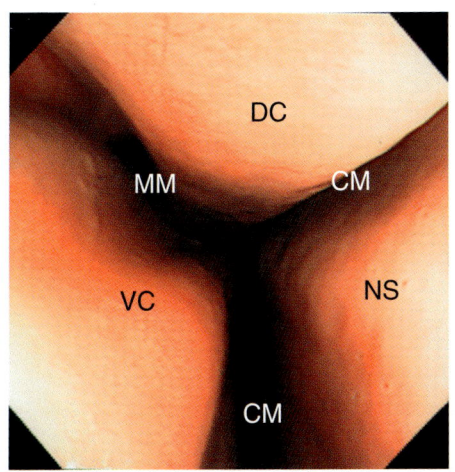

Fig. 3-4: Middle (MM) and common (CM) nasal meatuses of the right nasal cavity in the normal horse. The middle meatus is defined as the space between the dorsal and ventral conchae, and the common meatus is the space between the conchae and the nasal septum – note the 'y'-shape created by the dorsal concha (DC) dorsally, the ventral concha (VC) ventro-laterally and the nasal septum (NS) medially. The lateral part of the middle meatus is usually too small to pass an endoscope into.

The caudal aspect of the nasal cavities should be examined in detail because there are several structures of clinical significance located here; the ethmoturbinates and the communication with the paranasal sinuses (known as the sinus drainage angle) are both situated at the caudal aspect of the middle meatus (Fig. 3-6).

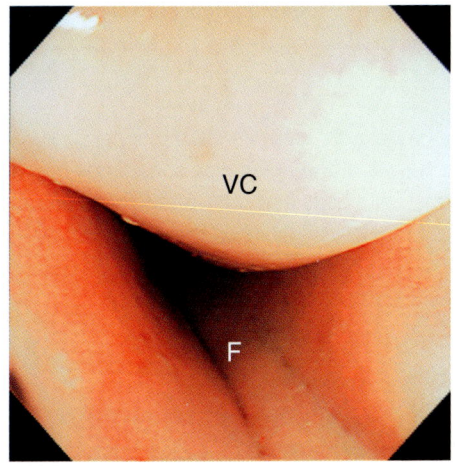

Fig. 3-5: Ventral nasal meatus of the right nasal cavity in the normal horse. This is the largest of the nasal meatuses and is a 'u'-shape, created by the ventral aspect of the ventral nasal concha dorsally (VC) and the floor of the nasal cavities ventrally (F).

Handbook of Equine Respiratory Endoscopy

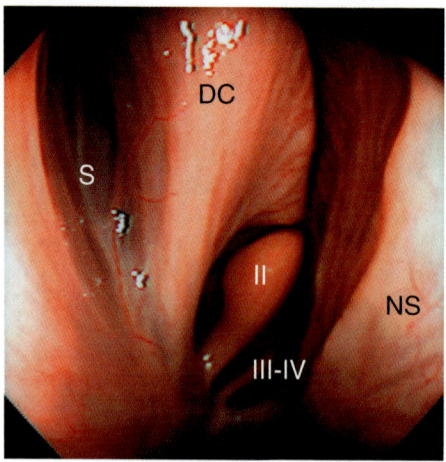

Fig. 3-6: Caudal aspect of the middle meatus showing the sinus drainage angle (S), dorsal concha (DC), nasal septum (NS), endoturbinate II and endoturbinates III–IV (II, III–IV).

Tips for endoscopic examination

The ventral meatus is quite large and is therefore most often used for passage of endoscopes, stomach tubes etc. into the nasopharynx and beyond. To perform endoscopy of the middle, common and dorsal meatuses, a small diameter scope (e.g. 8 mm diameter) should be used to avoid traumatizing the nasal mucosa. The mucosal lining of the nasal cavities is very vascular, and may bleed if it is accidentally traumatized by the tip of the endoscope (Fig. 3-7). If the endoscope is passed along the middle meatus, the ethmoturbinates and sinus drainage angle will naturally come into view (Fig. 3-6). To view this area with the endoscope passed up the ventral meatus, the endoscopist should simply direct the endoscope dorsally when the tip of the endoscope approaches the entrance to the nasopharynx.

If a large intraluminal mass (e.g. a neoplasm or ethmoidal hematoma) obstructs passage of the endoscope within the nasal cavity, the caudal aspect of the mass may sometimes be visualized by passing the endoscope up the contralateral nostril and then retroflexing the tip of the scope after it has entered the nasopharynx, to look rostrally down the affected nasal cavity (Fig. 3-8).

Abnormalities

Extraluminal narrowing of the nasal cavities

This is most commonly caused by a space-occupying mass (e.g. sinus cyst or neoplasm) or accumulation of pus in the ipsilateral paranasal sinuses. Passage of the endoscope up the

Chapter 3: **Nasal cavities**

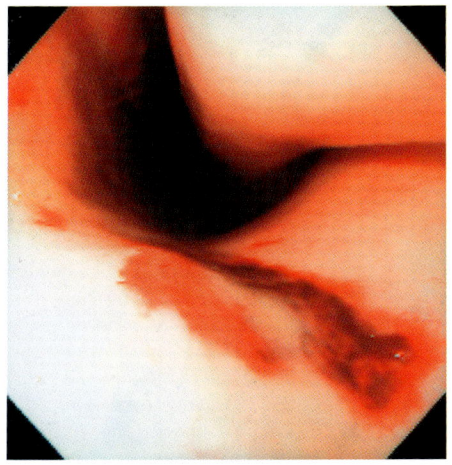

Fig. 3-7: Traumatic damage to the mucosa of the ventral meatus. This type of injury is commonly iatrogenic, occurring during nasogastric intubation, particularly if this procedure is repeated on several occasions. The horse can experience considerable epistaxis from damage to a small area of mucosa such as this.

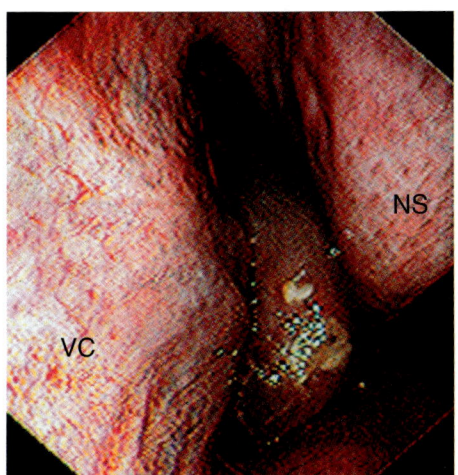

Fig. 3-8: Large intranasal progressive ethmoidal hematoma which completely prevented passage of the endoscope along the affected nasal cavity. The endoscope has been passed up the contralateral (right) nasal cavity and retroflexed back to face rostrally once it entered the nasopharynx in order to get this photograph which shows the caudal extent of the mass. NS = caudal aspect of the nasal septum, VC = ventral concha. Photograph courtesy of J. Perkins.

middle, common and/or ventral meatuses may be completely impeded by medial distension of the ventral conchal sinus (within the ventral concha) (Fig. 3-9). Occasionally, a disease process involving the dorsal conchal sinus may cause distortion of the dorsal concha and obliteration of the dorsal, common and middle meatuses. Radiography and sinoscopy (see Chapter 9) assist in determining the cause of sinus distension, and treatment must be directed at the cause of sinusitis.

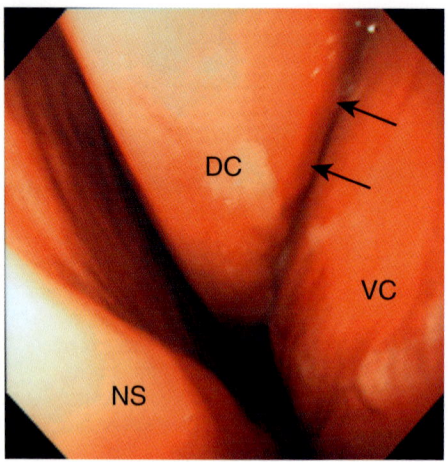

Fig. 3-9: Ventral conchal distention. Left nasal cavity of a horse with a sinus cyst within its ventral conchal sinus. Note how the lumen of the middle meatus (arrows) has been occluded by distension of the ventral concha (VC) which contains the expansive mass. DC = dorsal concha. NS = nasal septum.

Nasal mycosis (Fig. 3-10)

Primary mycotic infections of the equine nasal cavities are uncommon but nasal mycosis often occurs secondary to other disorders, such as sinusitis, nasal neoplasia, or traumatic damage to the nasal mucosa. Affected horses present with malodorous unilateral or bilateral nasal discharge or epistaxis. Primary mycotic infections can be very destructive, resulting in erosion of the nasal conchae (Fig. 9-22). If nasal mycosis is secondary to another disease process, resolution will usually occur when the primary problem is treated. Topical application of fungicidal solution (e.g. natamycin or enilconazole) to primary lesions, along with gentle debridement of loose plaques usually results in a favorable response.

Rhinitis sicca

This is a particular feature of grass sickness (equine dysautonomia). Affected horses may make adventitious respiratory noises and olfaction is adversely affected, resulting in anorexia and a worse prognosis for severely affected cases. Dry crusty plaques and mucosal inflammation and ulceration are observed during endoscopic examination of the nasal cavities. No specific treatment is available for horses affected with rhinitis sicca.

Nasal polyps (Fig. 3-11)

The term nasal 'polyp' is not a definitive description of a particular lesion or disease process, but is used to describe a mass which protrudes from the nasal mucosa. Polyps may be pedunculated (attached via a thin stalk) or sessile (attached by a broad base) and may be inflammatory or neoplastic in origin. If large, they may obstruct nasal airflow.

Chapter 3: **Nasal cavities**

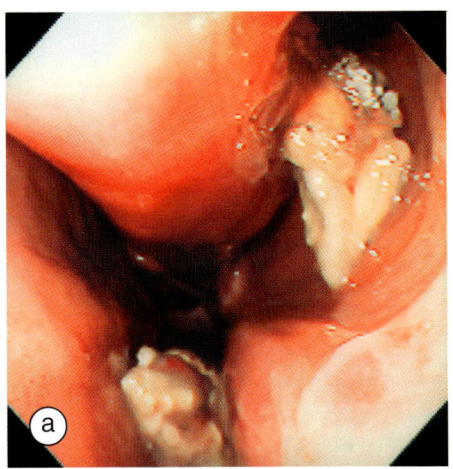

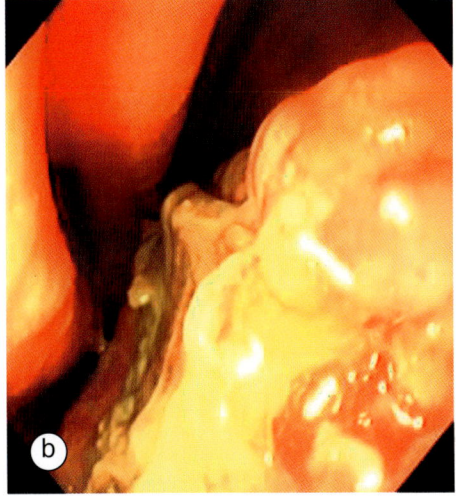

Fig. 3-10a, b: Fungal plaques typical of infection of the nasal cavities with *Aspergillus* spp. Note the 'moldy cheese' appearance of these lesions. The mucosa underlying these plaques is often ulcerated and bleeds easily.

Histological examination of biopsy samples taken from polyps should confirm their etiology. They can often be removed using a transendoscopic method such as laser surgery or electrosurgical snaring, or alternatively, an open surgical approach (e.g. nasal osteotomy) can be used.

Handbook of Equine Respiratory Endoscopy

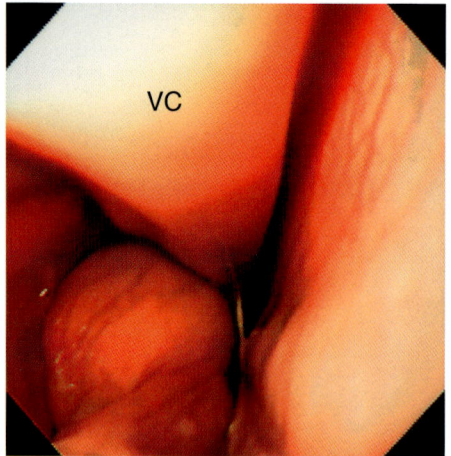

Fig. 3-11: Inflammatory polyp present in the nasal cavity of a horse with chronic sinusitis. The polyp is covered with normal respiratory mucosa and is causing partial obstruction of the ventral meatus. VC = ventral concha.

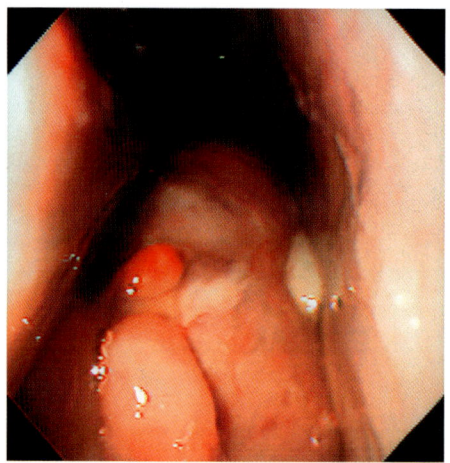

Fig. 3-12: Large lymphosarcoma obstructing the ventral meatus of a 20-year-old horse which presented with abnormal respiratory noise at rest and unilateral nasal discharge.

Neoplasia of the nasal cavities

Primary neoplasms of the nasal cavities are rare, but most frequently occur in older horses and are usually malignant. Adenocarcinoma, lymphosarcoma (Fig. 3-12), squamous cell carcinoma or osteogenic sarcoma are the most common tumor types. Clinical signs consist initially of unilateral purulent nasal discharge caused by mucosal inflammation and secondary bacterial infection. They often progress to unilateral obstruction of nasal airflow,

Chapter 3: **Nasal cavities**

lymphadenopathy, and facial swelling and may eventually extend to involve the contralateral side of the head. Endoscopy may reveal a mass or masses within the nasal cavity, but biopsy and histopathological examination will be required to make a definitive diagnosis and hence plan a treatment strategy if possible.

Apical infection of the rostral maxillary cheek teeth

Periapical infections of the rostral two maxillary cheek teeth (upper 06's and 07's, Triadan system) most commonly cause focal facial swelling and cutaneous draining tracts due to lateral extension of infection into the maxillary bone. Occasionally apical infections burst medially into the rostro-lateral aspect of the nasal cavity (Fig. 3-13a). Young horses are most commonly affected, and the tract is therefore often situated within the middle meatus, which is at the level of the apices of the long cheek teeth (Fig. 3-1). The tract is usually not visible using endoscopy, because most of the middle meatus is very narrow, but purulent discharge can be seen emanating from the rostral aspect of the middle meatus, with little or no discharge present further caudally in the nasal cavity. In older horses, periapical infection is often secondary to deep periodontal disease, and in such cases, the draining tract may be seen in the ventral nasal meatus, due to the relatively shorter length of reserve crown in these animals. Food material that has migrated up the diseased periodontal space and through the oronasal fistula may also be noted in the nasal cavity (Fig. 3-13b). The oral cavity should be examined using a full mouth speculum (gag) to identify periodontal disease or other dental abnormalities. Definitive diagnosis of periapical infection requires radiographic examination of the affected tooth apex. Scintigraphic examination of the skull

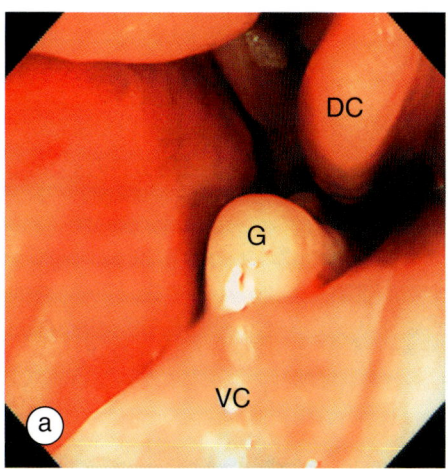 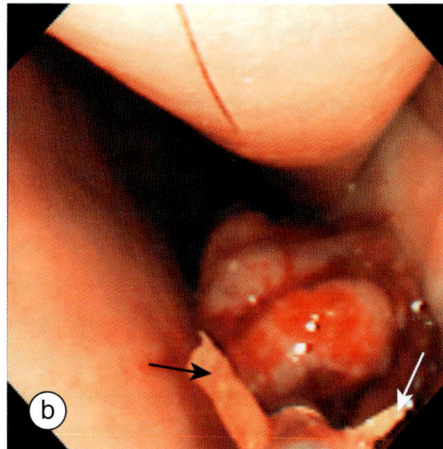

Fig. 3-13: Periapical infection of cheek teeth.
a) Middle meatus of a 7-year-old horse with a chronic periapical abscess of 107 which caused both facial swelling and a unilateral nasal discharge. There is marked erosion and remodeling of the dorsal concha (DC) with infected granulation tissue present (G), and some deformity of the ventral concha (VC).
b) Granuloma and food material (arrows) in the ventral meatus. This horse had periapical infection of 207 secondary to a complete, displaced sagittal fracture of this tooth with food impacted between the two dental fragments.

may be useful when radiographic changes are equivocal. Treatment usually involves extraction of the tooth (*per os*, by repulsion or by lateral buccotomy), and sealing of the oronasal fistula.

Progressive ethmoidal hematomas (Figs 3-14a, b)

A progressive ethmoidal hematoma (PEH) is a hemorrhagic lesion of unknown etiopathogenesis, usually originating from the submucosa of the ethmoidal labyrinth at the caudal aspect of the middle meatus. They may grow rostrally into the nasal cavity, and/or caudally into the nasopharynx. They can occur bilaterally, and therefore in horses with suspected or confirmed PEH, both nasal cavities should be examined endoscopically. Affected horses are usually presented because of chronic, intermittent, low-grade, serosanguinous nasal discharge. A PEH is easily identified by its characteristic dark red/brown/greenish color when visualized endoscopically (Fig. 3-14a). Occasionally a PEH may originate on the dorsal or lateral aspects of the ethmoturbinates, within the paranasal sinuses (see Chapter 9), and in such cases, hemorrhagic discharge may be seen emanating from the sinus drainage angle. Treatment most commonly involves transendoscopic injection of the PEH with 10% formalin (Fig. 3-14b) on several occasions, which results in necrosis of the lesion (Fig. 3-14c). Laser ablation or open surgical resection are also used by some clinicians.

Discharges from, or abnormalities of, the sinus drainage angle

Endoscopic examination *per nasum* of horses affected with paranasal sinusitis usually reveals an abnormal discharge emanating from the sinus drainage angle in the caudal aspect of the middle meatus (Fig. 3-15). This finding is an indication for radiographic and possibly sinoscopic examination of the affected sinuses (see Chapter 9). When a specific diagnosis is confirmed, appropriate treatment can then be instigated.

The sino-nasal ostium is slit-like in most normal horses, and therefore does not facilitate direct sinus endoscopy. In horses that have previously undergone sinus surgery with sino-nasal fistulation (to improve drainage from the sinuses), a large opening usually persists at this site (Fig. 3-16). This fistula may be large enough to accommodate the endoscope, allowing direct inspection of the paranasal sinuses. Occasionally, horses with chronic infection of the paranasal sinuses may have a large sino-nasal opening without any history of surgery being performed – this is presumably due to an erosive process such as mycotic infection (Fig. 9-22) or a large abscess 'bursting' through the medial wall of the sinus into the nasal cavity. The sino-nasal ostium may occasionally become deformed by an intrasinus mass (e.g. PEH) that has expanded from the sinuses into the nasal cavity via the nasomaxillary ostium.

Foreign bodies

Horses rarely inhale foreign bodies, but affected animals may present with a history of paroxysmal snorting followed by unilateral nasal discharge. Most nasal foreign bodies can be removed endoscopically using grasping or basket forceps (Fig. 3-17).

Chapter 3: **Nasal cavities**

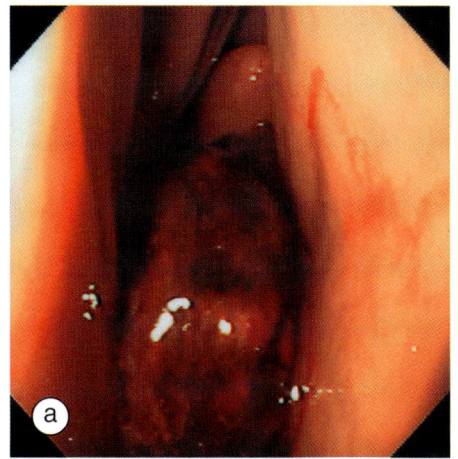

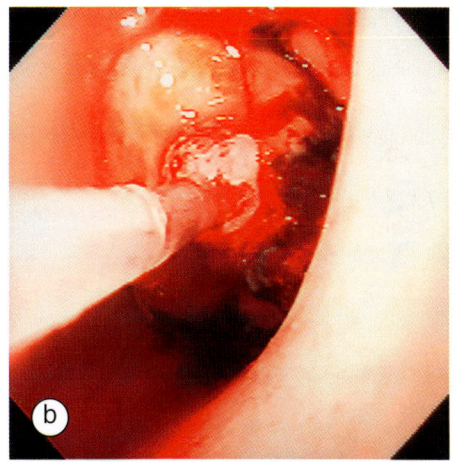

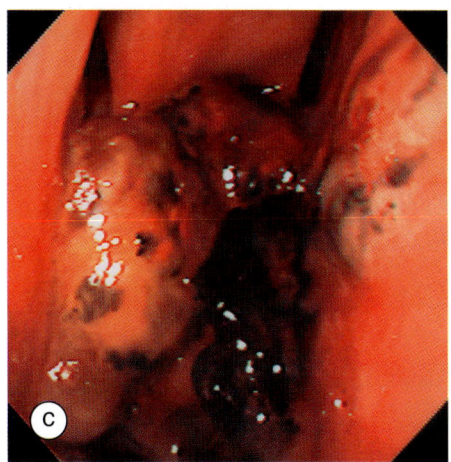

Fig. 3-14:
a) Progressive ethmoidal hematoma growing rostrally into the right nasal cavity from the ethmoidal region. Note the characteristic dark red-brown color.
b) This ethmoidal hematoma is being injected with formalin transendoscopically using a Teflon™ catheter which has been cut obliquely to give it a sharp leading edge (see Fig. 1-7) that is able to penetrate the soft hematoma.
c) Progressive ethmoidal hematoma 1 week after injection with formalin, showing slow disintegration of the lesion.

Handbook of Equine Respiratory Endoscopy

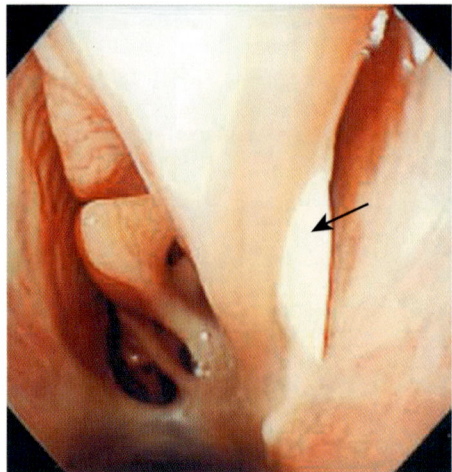

Fig. 3-15: Purulent material (arrow) emanating from the left sinus drainage angle of a horse with sinusitis.

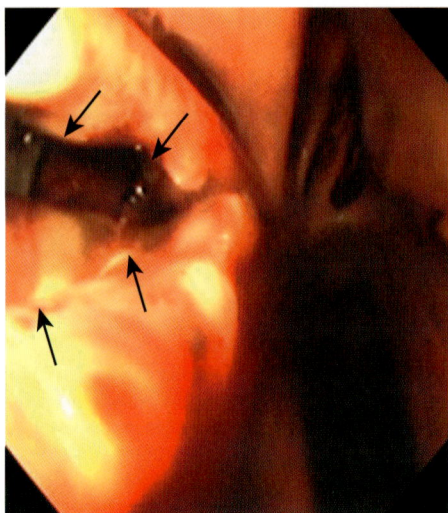

Fig. 3-16: Sino-nasal fistula. View of the caudal aspect of the middle meatus in a horse which underwent sinus flap surgery 5 days previously (the ethmoturbinates can be seen in the distance). A surgically created sino-nasal fistula (arrows) has been made in the dorso-medial aspect of the ventral concha through which the endoscope can now be passed to allow direct inspection of the sinus contents. Purulent material is draining from the sinus into the nasal cavity via this fistula.

Chapter 3: **Nasal cavities**

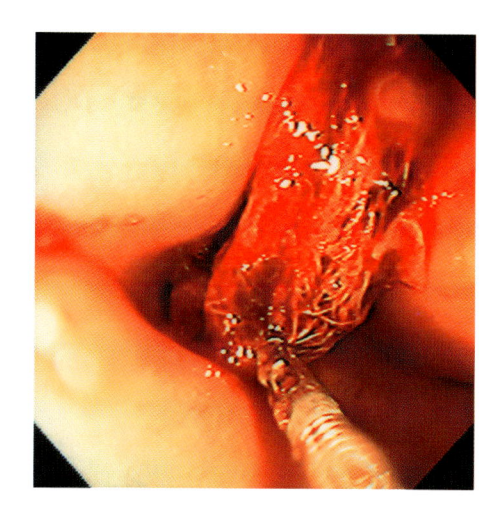

Fig. 3-17: Foreign body being retrieved from the nasal cavity using transendoscopic grasping forceps.

Nasal septum deviation

Nasal septum deviation is usually a congenital disorder, referred to as 'wry nose'. Foals with wry nose have gross lateral deviation of the maxillae, pre-maxillae, nasal bones and nasal septum. The condition can be variable in severity, and is externally obvious in most cases, as the nose is twisted to one side (Fig. 3-18). Endoscopically, the nasal cavities have a lateral 'curvature' which is noticeable as the endoscope is advanced towards the nasopharynx. Most mildly affected horses are able to perform all but the most strenuous activities (i.e. racing) successfully without recourse to surgery, although attention must be paid to management of dental disorders/overgrowths that occur with this condition. Surgical treatment to correct wry nose is extremely difficult, but removal of the nasal septum may restore respiratory capacity to near normal.

Occasionally, nasal septum deviation may be caused by a space-occupying lesion in one nasal cavity which pushes the cartilaginous nasal septum across the midline, thereby narrowing the contralateral nasal meatuses.

Choanal atresia (Fig. 3-19)

This is a rare congenital abnormality caused by persistence of the buccopharyngeal septum during embryonic development. If the disorder is bilateral, foals often asphyxiate shortly after birth before an emergency tracheostomy can be performed. Unilaterally affected horses may be asymptomatic at rest but may make a loud abnormal respiratory noise during exercise. No airflow is detected from the affected nostril, and endoscopic examination of the affected nasal cavity will reveal a membranous or bony septum at the caudal aspect of the nasal cavity that obstructs passage of the endoscope into the nasopharynx. Treatment involves removal of the abnormal septum.

Handbook of Equine Respiratory Endoscopy

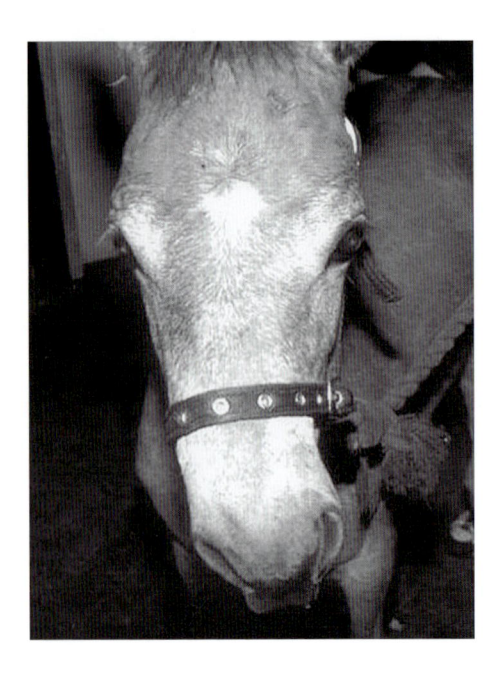

Fig. 3-18: Foal with wry nose. Note the marked deviation of the nose to the left due to shortening of the maxilla, pre-maxilla and nasal bones on this side. Photograph courtesy of P. Dixon.

Fig. 3-19: Choanal atresia. This horse has a thin membranous septum at the caudal extent of its left nasal cavity which prevents caudal passage of the endoscope into the nasopharynx.

Chapter 3: **Nasal cavities**

FURTHER READING

Dixon PM, Schumacher J 2006 Disorders of the nasal passages. In: Equine Respiratory Medicine and Surgery Eds: McGorum, Robinson, Schumacher and Dixon, Saunders

Head KW, Dixon PM 1999 Equine nasal and paranasal sinus tumours. Part 1: Review of the literature and tumour classification. Veterinary Journal 157:261–78

Nickels FA 1993 Diseases of the nasal cavity. Veterinary Clinic of North America, Equine Practice 9:111–21

Schumacher J, Yarbrough T, Pascoe J et al. 1998 Transendoscopic chemical ablation of progressive ethmoidal haematomas in standing horses. Veterinary surgery 27:175–81

Chapter preview

Normal anatomy 31

Tips for endoscopic examination 34

Abnormalities 35
    Pharyngeal lymphoid hyperplasia (PLH) 35
    Pharyngeal paralysis 36
    Nasopharyngeal collapse 37
    Secretions emanating from the guttural pouch ostia 37
    Pharyngeal accumulation of respiratory secretions 37
    Intermittent dorsal displacement of the soft palate (DDSP) 38
    Persistent dorsal displacement of the soft palate 40
    Cleft palate 41
    Iatrogenic palate defects 44
    Neoplasia 44
    Foreign bodies 44
    Palatal or pharyngeal cysts 46

Further reading 47

4: Pharynx

Normal anatomy (Figs 4-1 and 4-2)

The pharynx is a muscular tube that connects the nasal and oral cavities rostrally to the larynx and esophagus caudally. The horse has an intranarial larynx, with the cartilages of the larynx being 'locked' into the caudal wall of the nasopharynx by the palatopharyngeal arch. The muscular soft palate completely divides the nasopharynx from the oropharynx at all times except during swallowing. The nasopharynx is lined with mucosa beneath which lie visible submucosal blood vessels. The dorsal pharyngeal recess is positioned in the rostral aspect of the nasopharynx, and the mucosa in and surrounding this area contains a particularly high density of lymphatic tissue. Lymphatic tissue is additionally spread more diffusely in the mucosa of all other aspects of the nasopharynx.

The floor of the nasopharynx is formed by the dorsal aspect of the soft palate, which has longitudinal ridges that become more apparent when the palate is flaccid. Horses that resent endoscopic examination of the respiratory tract often tense the soft palate, giving its rostral aspect a dorsally 'domed' appearance (Fig. 4-3). The caudal border of the soft palate normally fits snugly around the base of the epiglottis (Fig. 4-4).

The guttural pouch ostia are cartilaginous flaps which lead to the auditory tubes and then the guttural pouches. They are positioned on the dorso-lateral walls of the rostral nasopharynx. The guttural pouches are situated dorsal to the roof of the caudal nasopharynx, and distension of the pouches can cause the roof of the nasopharynx to collapse.

The oropharynx is a small space, located caudal to the 6th cheek teeth, ventral to the soft palate and rostral to the epiglottis (Fig. 4-5). During normal breathing, the soft palate lies directly on the base of the tongue, and most of the oropharynx is therefore a 'potential'

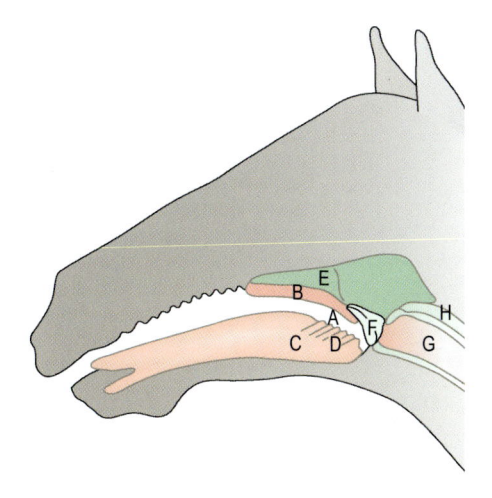

Fig. 4-1: Schematic diagram of the pharynx of the horse: A = oropharynx; B = soft palate; C = tongue; D = lingual tonsil; E = nasopharynx; F = epiglottis; G = trachea; H = esophagus.

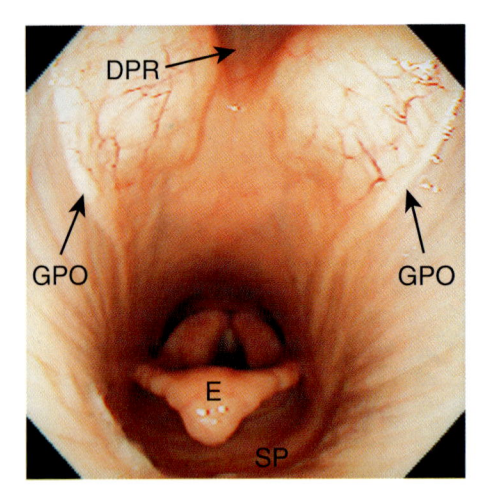

Fig. 4-2: Nasopharynx in the normal horse. The dorsal aspect of the soft palate (SP) forms the floor of the nasopharynx. The cartilaginous flaps of the guttural pouch ostia (GPO) lie on the dorso-lateral walls of the nasopharynx. The dorsal pharyngeal recess (DPR) is positioned in the midline in the rostral part of the nasopharyngeal roof. The epiglottic cartilage (E) should lie dorsal to the soft palate.

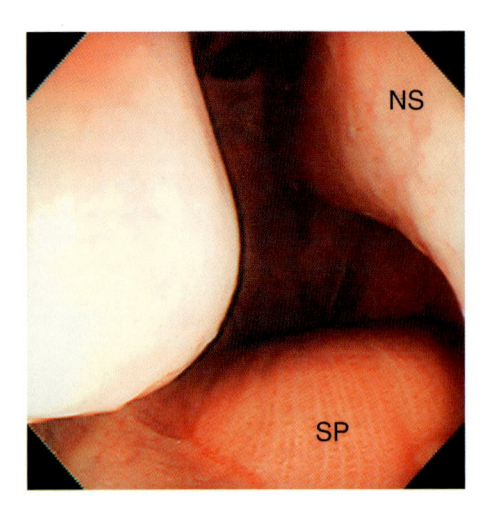

Fig. 4-3: Rostral aspect of the nasopharynx (viewed with the endoscope passed up the right nasal cavity) in a normal horse which resents endoscopy and has tensed its soft palate (SP), giving it a dorsally 'domed' appearance. Note the longitudinal ridges on the soft palate. The nasal septum (NS), which is incomplete at its caudal aspect, is just visible.

Chapter 4: Pharynx

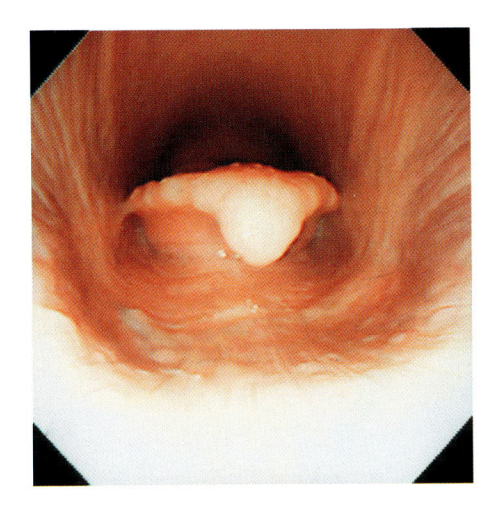

Fig. 4-4: Caudal aspect of the ventral nasopharynx showing the normal relationship between the soft palate and the epiglottis, with the caudal border of the soft palate fitting snugly around the base of the epiglottis. Small amounts of mucopurulent respiratory secretions are present on the floor of the nasopharynx.

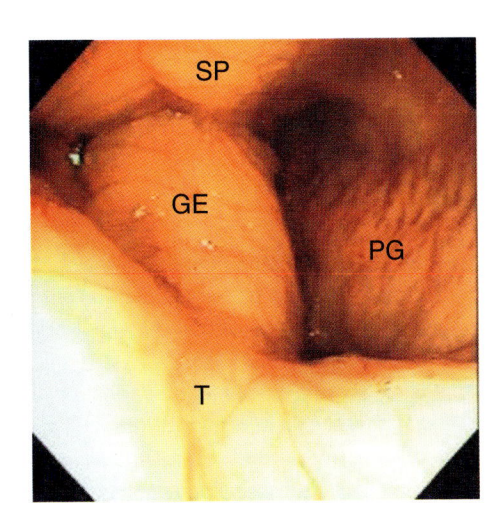

Fig. 4-5: Oropharynx in the normal horse. SP = soft palate, T = tongue, GE = glossoepiglottic (subepiglottic) folds, PG = left palatoglossal arch.

space, except during swallowing. The caudo-dorsal aspect of the tongue is covered with lymphatic tissue, termed the 'lingual tonsil', and has an uneven appearance. The hyoepiglottic muscles and ligaments connect the ventral aspect of the epiglottis to the base of the tongue and are covered by the glossoepiglottic mucosal fold. The palatoglossal arches form the lateral aspects of the oropharynx and connect the dorsal base of the tongue to the ventral aspect of the soft palate.

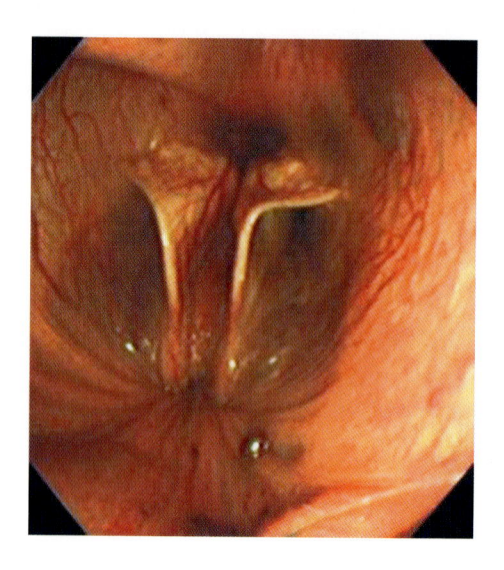

Fig. 4-6: Bilateral dilation of the guttural pouch ostia occurring during swallowing.

During swallowing, contraction of the muscles at the base of the tongue is followed by a wave of constriction of the circular muscles of the pharyngeal walls, which pushes ingesta to the caudal aspect of the oropharynx. This circular, caudally directed wave of constriction causes the guttural pouch ostia to dilate (Fig. 4-6). The soft palate then elevates and the epiglottis retroverts, allowing ingesta to flow over the adducted larynx into the esophagus.

In the normal horse, a small amount of mucoid respiratory secretions may be present on the walls of the nasopharynx, but food material should not be seen.

Tips for endoscopic examination

Endoscopic examination of the nasopharynx is performed by passing the endoscope *per nasum* as described in Chapter 2. Some clinicians occlude the nares during endoscopic examination to increase intrapharyngeal pressures and try to induce dorsal displacement of the soft palate (DDSP); however, the fact that DDSP occurs during nasal occlusion at rest is not an accurate predictor that the disorder occurs at exercise, and conversely, some horses that do not displace their palates during nasal occlusion at rest experience DDSP at exercise. Passage of the endoscope into the trachea often results in transient DDSP (viewed as the endoscope is withdrawn into the nasopharynx), but most horses will replace the soft palate immediately by swallowing, therefore this finding is usually insignificant.

Endoscopic examination of the oropharynx is most commonly indicated in cases where the soft palate is persistently dorsally displaced, obscuring visualization of the epiglottis. A full mouth speculum must be placed in the horse's mouth to protect the endoscope from trauma from the cheek teeth. A flexible endoscope can be guided to the oropharynx using an assistant's hand or a section of 5 cm diameter PVC pipe. The presence of the endoscope in the horse's mouth induces chewing/swallowing movements, which can make visualization of the oropharynx and epiglottis difficult. To minimize these movements, heavy sedation is usually required, and intravenous diazepam may also further reduce activity of the tongue.

Chapter 4: **Pharynx**

Abnormalities

Pharyngeal lymphoid hyperplasia (PLH)

Enlargement of the lymphoid follicles on the walls and roof of the nasopharynx and particularly around the dorsal pharyngeal recess is an extremely common finding in young horses (Fig. 4-7). PLH was previously believed to be associated with abnormal respiratory

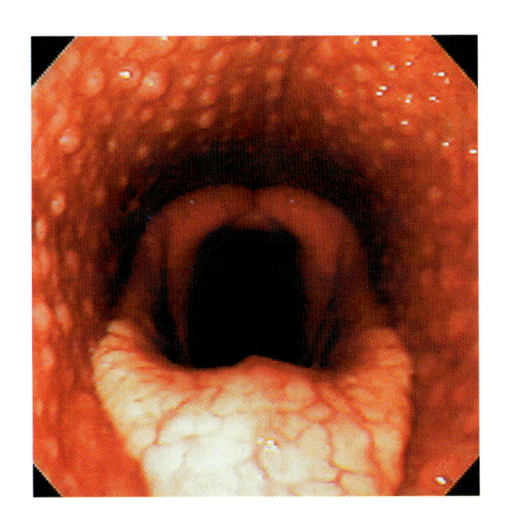

Fig. 4-7: Pharyngeal lymphoid hyperplasia in the nasopharynx of a 2-year-old Thoroughbred racehorse. Note the prominent lymphoid follicles on the lateral and dorsal pharyngeal walls. This finding is considered to be normal in young horses, and does not affect performance during exercise.

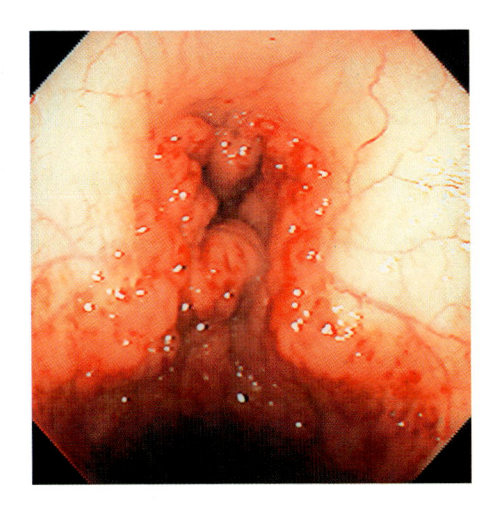

Fig. 4-8: Marked pharyngeal lymphoid hyperplasia concentrated around the dorsal nasopharyngeal recess associated with acute viral respiratory infection in a 9-year-old horse.

noise at exercise and blamed for poor performance, but the condition is now considered to be of little clinical significance in young horses. As the horse matures, these prominent follicles usually reduce in size. However, they can enlarge again if older horses are exposed to infectious respiratory agents (Fig. 4-8), or if some other pathological process (e.g. neoplasia) induces inflammation in the nasopharynx. A four-grade system has been developed to document the severity of PLH, based on the degree of hyperplasia and distribution of hyperplastic follicles within the nasopharynx, but it is not commonly used due to the majority of horses with PLH being clinically 'normal'. No treatment is indicated for horses with this condition. If PLH is secondary to some other disease process, treatment should be directed at the primary disorder.

Pharyngeal paralysis

The most common cause of pharyngeal paralysis or dysphagia is guttural pouch mycosis that has resulted in damage to the 9th, 10th or 11th cranial nerves, which innervate the pharyngeal plexus (see Chapter 5). Pharyngeal paralysis may also occur due to neuromuscular dysfunction caused by congenital disorders, heavy metal poisoning, hypocalcemia, botulism and grass sickness (equine dysautonomia). Occasionally, temporary functional pharyngeal paralysis may develop in horses infected with *Streptococcus equi* (strangles).

Affected horses present with bilateral nasal discharge containing saliva and food material, and sometimes signs of lower respiratory disease caused by inhalation of ingesta into the trachea and/or small airways. Endoscopically, food material and saliva are seen on the walls and floor of the nasal cavities, nasopharynx (Fig. 4-9), larynx and trachea. In severe cases,

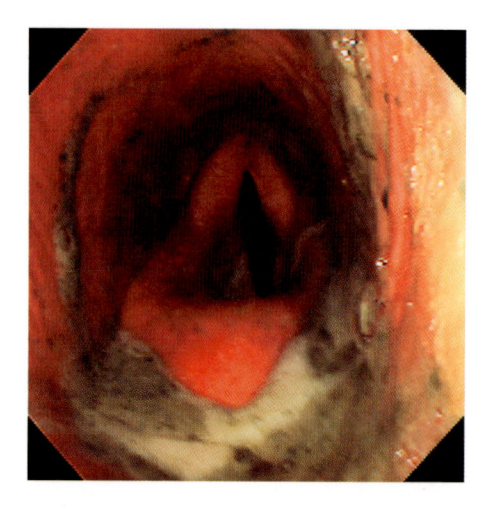

Fig. 4-9: Horse with pharyngeal paralysis secondary to guttural pouch mycosis. Note the food material on the walls of the nasopharynx and pooling of saliva and food on the floor of the pharynx. Left-sided recurrent laryngeal neuropathy is also present.

Chapter 4: **Pharynx**

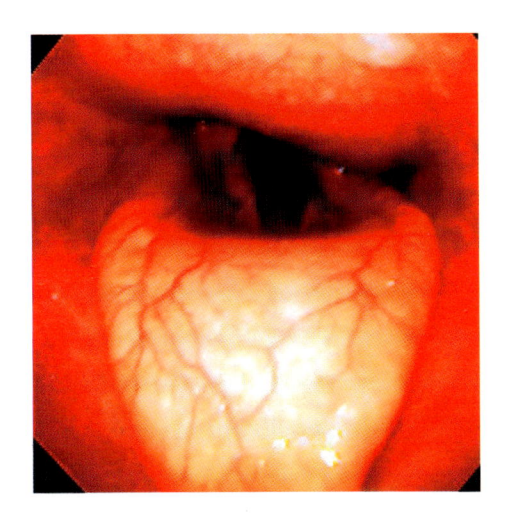

Fig. 4-10: Dorsal nasopharyngeal collapse (left side worse affected) due to a large melanoma growing in the left guttural pouch with metastasis to the retropharyngeal lymph nodes. Photograph courtesy of P. M. Dixon.

one or both sides of the nasopharynx may be collapsed. When the horse is stimulated to swallow (e.g. by spraying water down the biopsy channel of the endoscope), the circular constricting action of the pharyngeal muscles may be reduced or absent, and the guttural pouch ostia may not dilate. The soft palate may be persistently displaced.

There is no specific treatment for horses affected with pharyngeal paralysis. Treatment should be directed at resolving the primary disorder (e.g. guttural pouch mycosis), if one can be identified.

Nasopharyngeal collapse (Fig. 4-10)

Nasopharyngeal collapse may occur only during exercise or may be detected during endoscopy performed with the horse at rest. Dynamic nasopharyngeal collapse is discussed in more detail in Chapter 8. Collapse that is present in the resting horse is usually caused by disorders of the guttural pouches (e.g. melanomas, guttural pouch tympany or empyema) or marked enlargement of the retropharyngeal lymph nodes (associated with *Streptococcus equi* [strangles] infection). Occasionally, nasopharyngeal collapse can occur as a symptom of primary neuromuscular disease (e.g. botulism), and may be associated with pharyngeal paralysis.

Secretions emanating from the guttural pouch ostia (Fig. 4-11)

Disorders affecting the guttural pouches often result in abnormal secretions such as blood or purulent material emanating from the ostium of the affected guttural pouch(es). These disorders are discussed in more detail in Chapter 5.

Pharyngeal accumulation of respiratory secretions (Fig. 4-12)

Abnormal amounts of respiratory secretions observed on the walls or floor of the nasopharynx during endoscopy are most likely to be originating from the lower airways. Alternatively, secretions may flow caudally from the sinus drainage angle into the nasopharynx or may have emanated from the guttural pouches. Endoscopic examination of these other structures is warranted to ascertain the origin of the secretions.

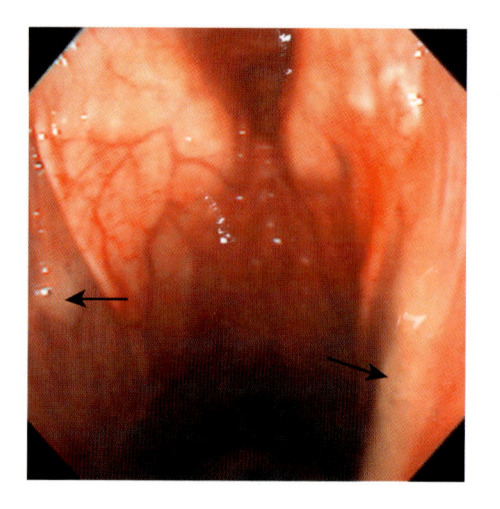

Fig. 4-11: Purulent material emanating from both guttural pouch ostia (arrows), in a case of guttural pouch empyema. This horse had an acute infection with *Streptococcus equi* (strangles).

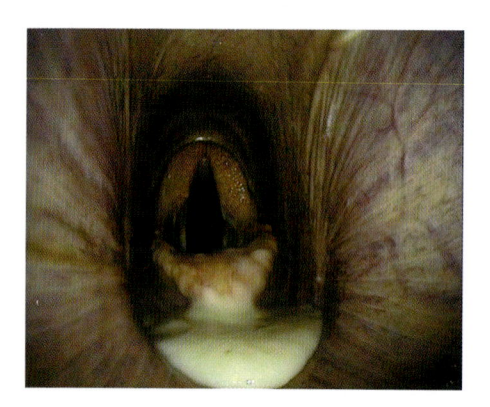

Fig. 4-12: Large amounts of thick purulent respiratory secretions accumulated on the floor of the nasopharynx in a horse with lower respiratory tract infection. Tracheoscopy revealed a pool of similar secretions at the level of the tracheal sump.

Intermittent dorsal displacement of the soft palate (DDSP)

Intermittent DDSP is a disorder that characteristically occurs in racehorses towards the end of fast work, when the caudal border of the soft palate becomes displaced dorsal to the epiglottis (Fig. 4-13). It is not possible to diagnose this condition during resting endoscopy. A definitive diagnosis of intermittent DDSP can currently only be made using high-speed treadmill endoscopy (see Chapter 8).

Chapter 4: **Pharynx**

Horses that have abnormalities of the palate or larynx, such as epiglottal entrapment, pharyngeal paralysis and palatal cysts, are predisposed to DDSP. In the absence of such abnormalities, the etiology of the disorder is currently unknown. It is likely to be multifactorial, but neuromuscular dysfunction of the intrinsic and/or extrinsic muscles of the soft palate may make a significant contribution to the development of this condition. Epiglottic hypoplasia or flaccidity was previously thought to be associated with intermittent DDSP. However, clinical and experimental data show that the epiglottis is not required to maintain the palate in a normal position, and that the majority of horses that are diagnosed with DDSP during treadmill endoscopy have an epiglottic length that is within normal limits. Some horses with intermittent DDSP have ulceration of the caudal border of the soft palate (Fig. 4-13b), and this is presumed to be caused by the unstable palate rubbing against the base of the epiglottis prior to displacement.

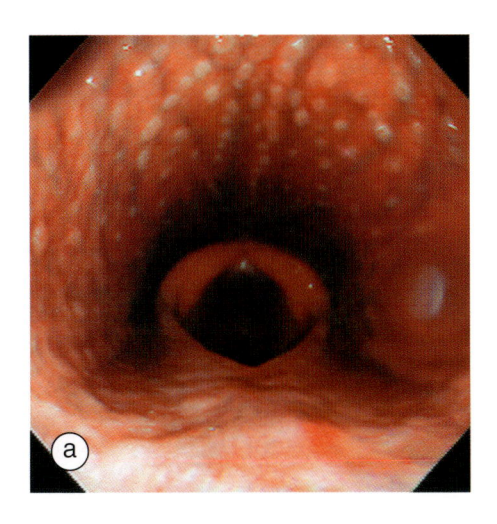

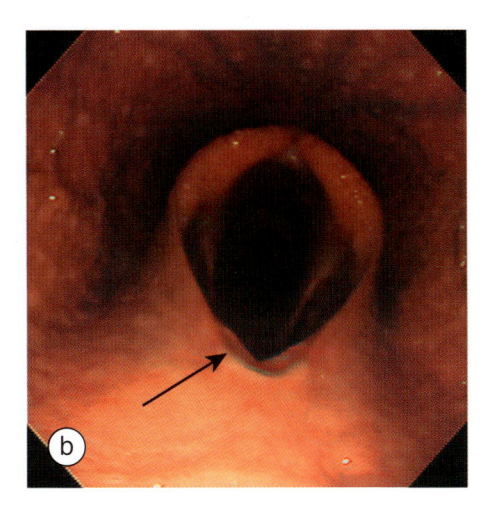

Fig. 4-13a, b: Dorsal displacement of the soft palate – photographs taken during high-speed treadmill endoscopy: the epiglottis can no longer be visualized due to the soft palate being displaced dorsal to it. In **b)** there is a small area of mucosal ulceration in the midline of the caudal border of the soft palate (arrow)

Most horses with DDSP make a 'gurgling' noise at exercise, which is attributable to the caudal edge of the displaced soft palate vibrating during respiration (Fig. 8-3), although some horses do not make any discernable abnormal respiratory noise. The displaced soft palate can almost completely obstruct the rima glottidis, and most affected horses will pull up abruptly or slow down significantly after the palate has displaced.

Many treatments are available for horses with DDSP, and this probably reflects both the unknown etiology of the disorder and the fact that most treatments have a similar success rate. Conservative remedies include rest, improvement of fitness, use of a tongue tie or dropped/crossed noseband, and systemic or topical medical therapy to encourage resolution of upper airway inflammation. Surgical treatments are numerous and include insertion of a thyrohyoid prosthesis (the 'tie-forward' or 'laryngo-hyoid reduction' procedure), staphylectomy, myectomy of the sternothyrohyoideus muscles, epiglottic augmentation with Teflon™, tension palatoplasty, thermocautery of the oral surface of the palate, and laser cautery of the nasopharyngeal surface of the palate (Fig. 4-14).

Persistent dorsal displacement of the soft palate

This disorder is rare, compared with intermittent DDSP, and usually occurs secondary to pharyngeal or laryngeal disorders that prevent the larynx from maintaining its normal intranarial position. It can occasionally be 'idiopathic'. Primary disorders associated with persistent DDSP include subepiglottic cysts, epiglottitis, epiglottic entrapment, intrapalatal cysts, pharyngeal paralysis, pharyngeal neoplasia and pharyngeal foreign bodies. Persistent DDSP may also be observed following epiglottic, pharyngeal or laryngeal surgery, particularly after surgery to release epiglottal entrapment if a large fold of the subepiglottic mucosa is resected. Horses affected with persistent DDSP make a loud gurgling noise at exercise, have poor exercise tolerance, and are often dysphagic.

If DDSP is persistent, the epiglottis is not visible with the endoscope passed *per nasum*, because the soft palate lies dorsal to it (Fig. 4-15). Ulceration of the caudal border of the soft palate can sometimes be observed. Observation of persistent DDSP with the scope passed *per nasum* is an indication to perform endoscopy of the oropharynx to examine the epiglottis and associated structures for abnormalities (Fig. 4-16a, b).

In most cases, persistent DDSP is secondary to some other disorder, and treatment should therefore be directed at the initiating cause. Insertion of a thyrohyoid prosthesis (the 'tie-forward' procedure) +/– laser staphylectomy has been reported to be effective in some cases of idiopathic persistent DDSP.

Chapter 4: **Pharynx**

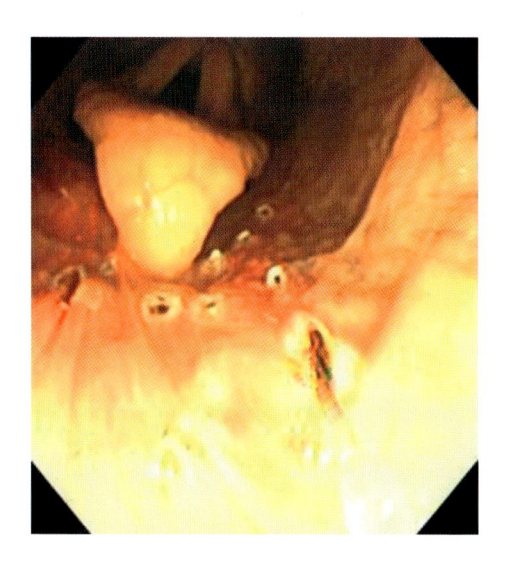

Fig. 4-14: Laser cautery of the soft palate. Note the multiple laser treatment points visible on the nasal aspect of the soft palate.

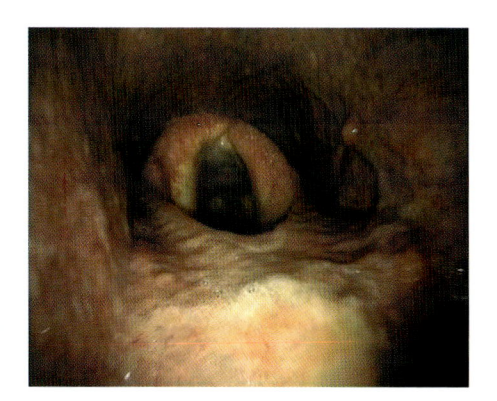

Fig. 4-15: Persistent DDSP. The epiglottic cartilage is no longer visible because it is lying ventral to the soft palate. The horse could not replace its palate, even after swallowing.

Cleft palate (Fig. 4-17)

Congenital defects of the palate are rare. They arise from abnormal embryological closure of the palatal folds, and defects may involve only the soft palate, or both the hard and soft palates. Affected foals should be examined carefully for other congenital defects. Clinical signs of cleft palate include nasal regurgitation of milk, coughing, and other clinical signs indicative of aspiration pneumonia. If the cleft is small, abnormal respiratory noise due to palatal instability or DDSP may be the only presenting sign.

Handbook of Equine Respiratory Endoscopy

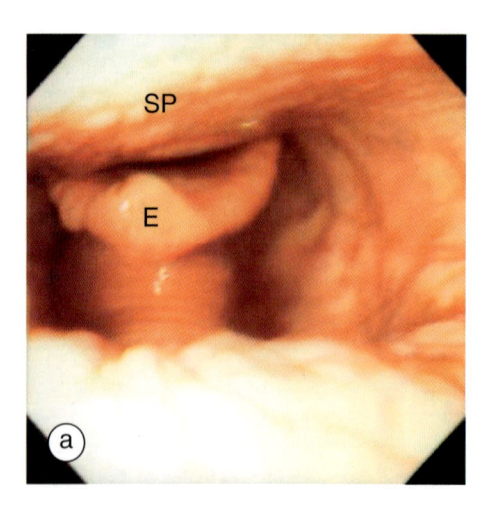

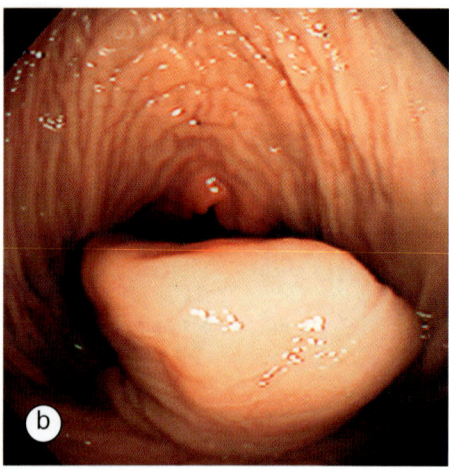

Fig. 4-16:

a) Oropharynx of a horse with idiopathic persistent DDSP. The epiglottic tip (E) appears slightly misshapen and is positioned ventral to the soft palate (SP), within the oropharynx.

b) Oropharynx of a horse with persistent DDSP secondary to epiglottal entrapment. Note that the epiglottic margin has lost its normally thin, serrated edge and appears rounded and thickened due to entrapment in the glossoepiglottic folds. Photograph courtesy of P. M. Dixon.

Endoscopic examination of the foal (using a small-diameter endoscope) reveals an abnormal outline to the caudal border of the soft palate, and food material within the nasopharynx, larynx and trachea. The only treatment available for foals with cleft palates is surgical repair, but this is a salvage procedure only, and most horses are unable to perform athletically even if surgery is successful. Surgical repair of soft palate defects has a high incidence of complications and failure, and euthanasia of affected foals should be considered as an alternative.

Chapter 4: **Pharynx**

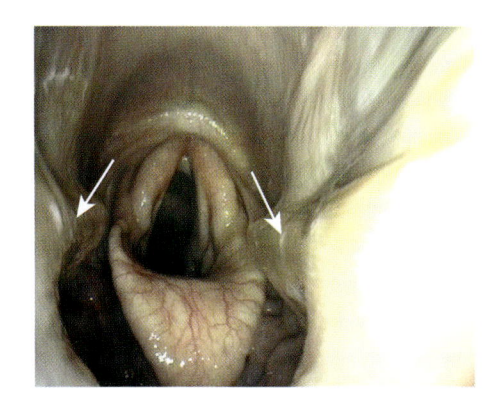

Fig. 4-17: Severe cleft palate. The lateral borders of the caudal palate are marked with arrows.

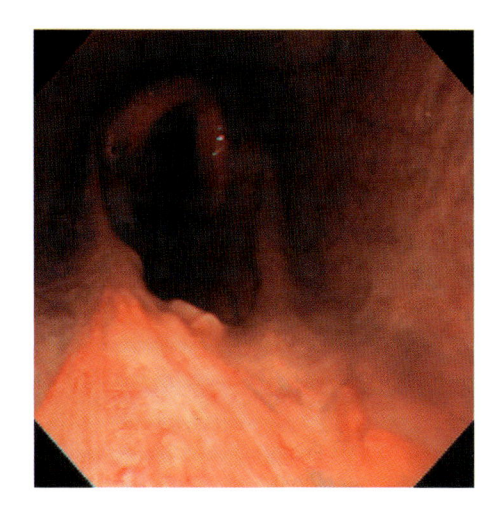

Fig. 4-18: This racehorse had previously had a staphylectomy for treatment of DDSP, during which too much tissue was removed from the left side of the caudal border of the palate. The soft palate is now persistently displaced, and the prognosis for a return to athletic function is very poor. Left recurrent laryngeal neuropathy is also present.

Iatrogenic palate defects (Fig. 4-18)

Defects of the soft palate may occur after staphylectomy if an excessive amount of tissue has been removed, after surgical removal of palatal lesions such as palatal cysts, or inadvertently during trans-nasal surgical correction of epiglottic entrapment using a hooked bistoury. Thermal, laser or excisional palatoplasty (performed as a treatment for intermittent DDSP) may also result in an oropharyngeal fistula if the full thickness of the palate is inadvertently damaged. Horses with iatrogenic palate defects may be dysphagic with nasal return of food or may simply have exacerbated signs of DDSP at exercise. Surgical correction of such lesions is difficult and affected horses have a guarded prognosis for return to full athletic function.

Neoplasia

Neoplasms of the nasopharynx are rare. Lymphosarcoma occurs most frequently and lesions may vary in appearance (Figs 4-19 and 4-20). Surgical excision of pharyngeal neoplasms is rarely successful, because surgical access is difficult and total excision with wide margins is almost impossible to achieve. Radiotherapy may provide an alternative for treatment of pharyngeal neoplasms, but is not widely available for horses.

Foreign bodies (Fig. 4-21)

Horses rarely inhale or ingest foreign bodies, but horses with a nasopharyngeal foreign body may present with dysphagia, stridor and nasal discharge, due to inflammation and secondary bacterial infection of the pharyngeal mucosa. Foreign bodies can usually be removed under endoscopic guidance using grasping or basket forceps or digitally *per os*.

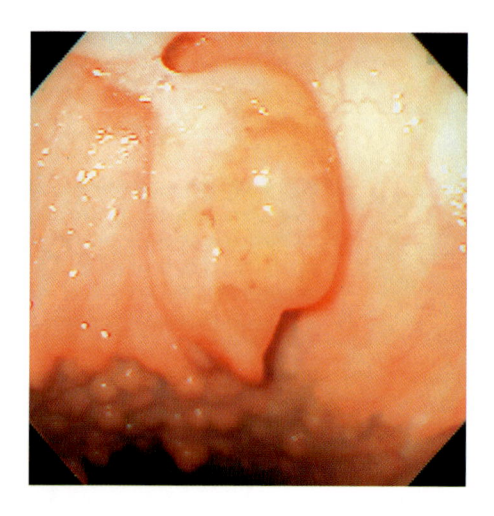

Fig. 4-19: Lymphosarcoma in the dorsal aspect of the pharynx in a 20-year-old horse. Note the prominent pharyngeal lymphoid hyperplasia which is present caudal to this lesion. Photograph courtesy of P. M. Dixon.

Chapter 4: **Pharynx**

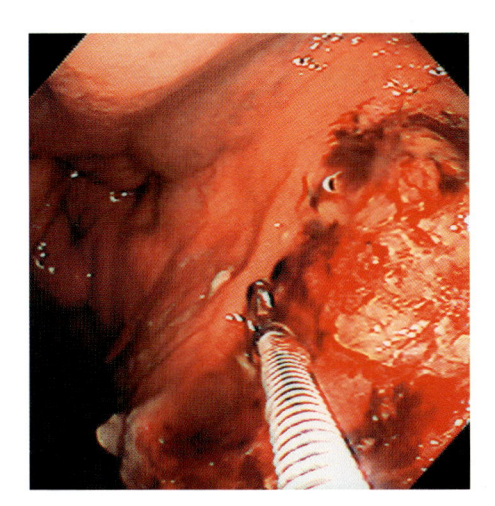

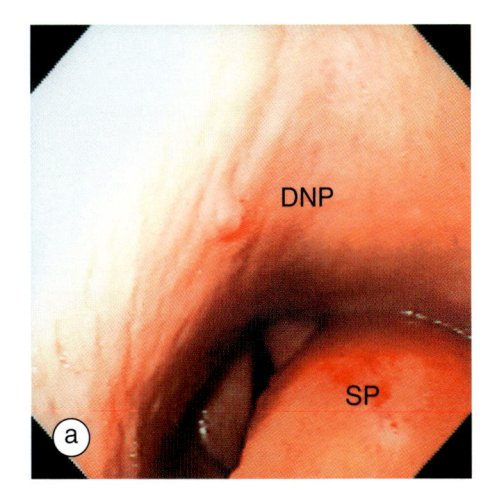

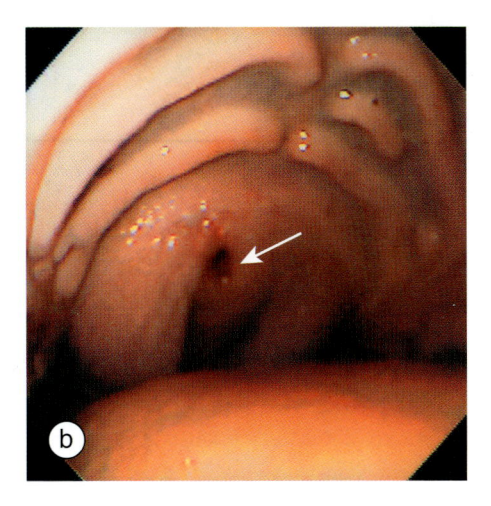

Fig. 4-20: Ulcerative lesion on the left lateral wall of the nasopharynx which is being biopsied transendoscopically. Histopathology revealed this to be a lymphosarcoma.

Fig. 4-21: Intrapalatal foreign body. This horse presented with severe stridor and progressive dyspnea.
a) Endoscopy *per nasum* revealed that the left caudal aspect of the soft palate (SP) was either markedly enlarged or was being pushed dorsally by a structure in the oropharynx, causing almost complete obstruction of the rima glottidis. DNP = dorsal nasopharynx.
b) Endoscopy *per os* (with a full mouth speculum in place) revealed a draining tract (arrow) in the rostral aspect of the soft palate, presumably caused by penetration of a foreign body.

45

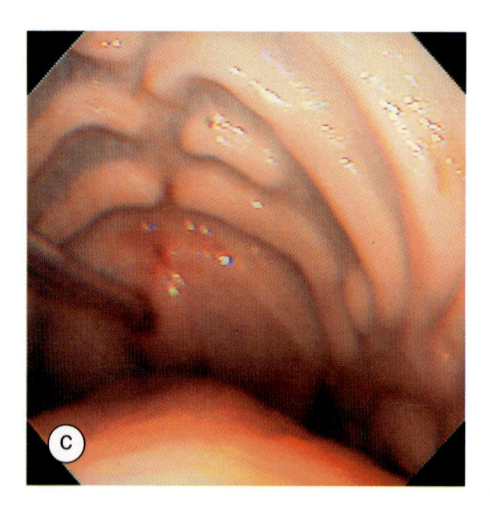

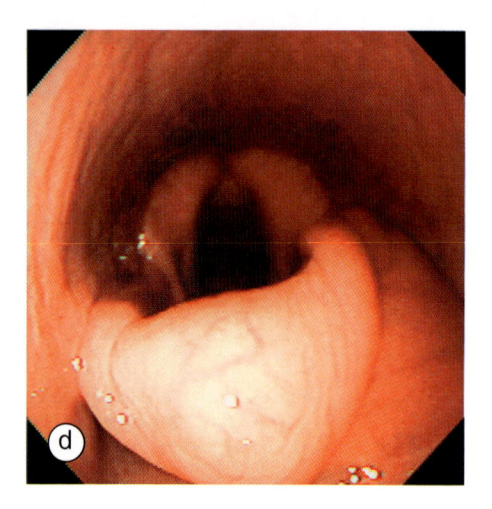

Fig. 4-21: *continued*

c) Forceps could be passed easily into this tract for a length of approximately 10 cm. No foreign body could be found within the tract/abscess. A tracheotomy tube was placed and the abscess left to drain into the mouth.

d) After 6 days, the size of the abscess in the soft palate had reduced markedly, and the tracheotomy tube was removed. The left side of the palate was still swollen, but this resolved completely over the following week.

Palatal or pharyngeal cysts

These rare lesions may be a cause of abnormal respiratory noise and airway obstruction if they become large. Pharyngeal cysts that are situated on the midline of the roof of the pharynx, caudal to the dorsal pharyngeal recess (Fig. 4-22) are thought to be remnants of Rathke's pouch (a diverticulum of the embryonic buccal cavity, from which the anterior lobe of pituitary gland is developed). The presence of palatal cysts predisposes horses to DDSP. Treatment involves surgical excision of the cystic structure, if it is large enough to cause abnormal respiratory noise or airway obstruction.

Chapter 4: **Pharynx**

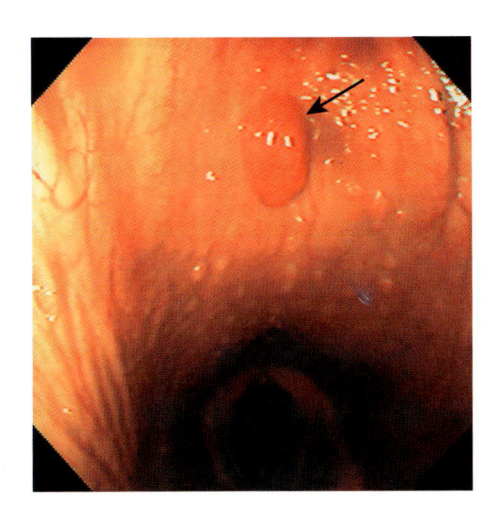

Fig. 4-22: Pharyngeal cyst (arrow) in the nasopharynx of a 5-year-old Thoroughbred located in the midline on the dorsal pharyngeal wall. This lesion is unlikely to be clinically significant, because it is too small to cause respiratory obstruction or turbulent airflow through the nasopharynx.

FURTHER READING

Holcombe SJ, Ducharme NG 2006 Disorders of the nasopharynx and soft palate. In: Equine Respiratory Medicine and Surgery. Eds: McGorum, Robinson, Schumacher and Dixon. Saunders

Holcombe SJ, Derksen FJ, Stick JA, Robinson NE 1999 Pathophysiology of dorsal displacement of the soft palate in horses. Equine Veterinary Journal Supplement 30:45–8

Parente EJ, Martin BB, Tulleners EP, et al. 2002 Dorsal displacement of the soft palate in 92 horses during high-speed treadmill examination (1993–1998). Veterinary Surgery 31:507–12

Sullivan EK, Parente EJ 2003 Disorders of the pharynx. Veterinary Clinics of North America Equine Practice 19:159–67

Chapter preview

Normal anatomy 49

Tips for endoscopic examination 53

Abnormalities 55

    Guttural pouch mycosis (GPM) 55

    Guttural pouch empyema 57

    Chondroids 59

    Guttural pouch tympany 61

    Neoplasia 62

    Temporohyoid osteopathy 63

    Rupture of the rectus capitus and longus capitus muscles 63

Further reading 64

5: Guttural pouches

Normal anatomy (Fig. 5-1)

The guttural pouches are large mucosa-lined outpouchings of the auditory (Eustachian) tubes which connect the nasopharynx to the middle ear. In a 500 kg horse they are around 350 cc in volume. The pouches are bordered dorsally by the base of the skull and the first cervical vertebra, ventrally by the retropharyngeal lymph nodes and the pharynx, dorso-medially by the rectus and longus capitus muscles, ventro-medially by a thin median septum and laterally by the pterygoid muscles and parotid and mandibular salivary glands.

Each pouch is incompletely divided into lateral and medial compartments by the stylohyoid bone (Fig. 5-2). This bone, which forms part of the hyoid apparatus, articulates dorsally with

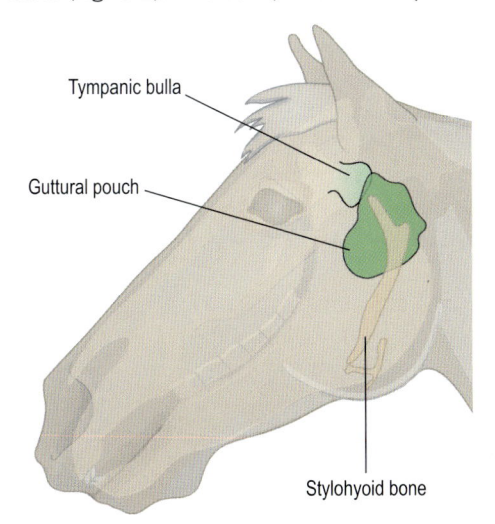

Fig. 5-1: Diagram of the position of the guttural pouch in the equine head showing its relation to the hyoid bones and tympanic bulla.

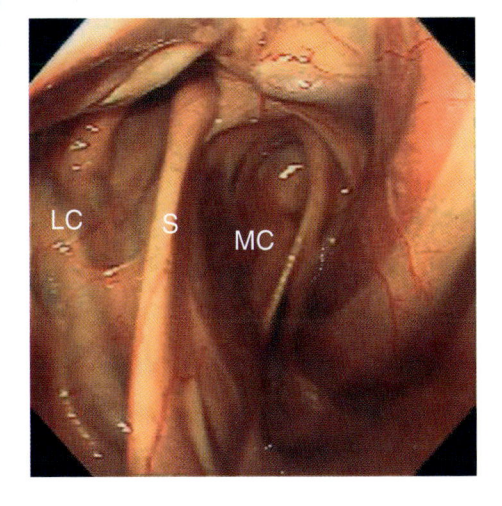

Fig. 5-2: Endoscopic view of the normal right guttural pouch. The stylohyoid bone (S) runs dorso-ventrally and incompletely separates the smaller lateral compartment (LC) from the large medial compartment (MC).

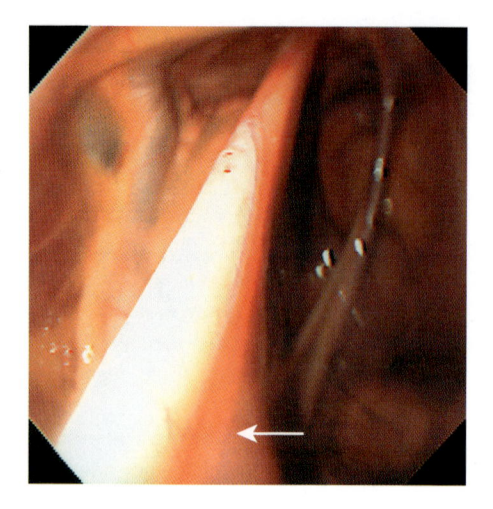

Fig. 5-3: Close-up view of the ventral aspect of the stylohyoid bone showing attachment of the stylopharyngeus muscle (arrow).

the petrous temporal bone at the base of the skull (i.e. the temporo-hyoid articulation), and ventrally, with the keratohyoid bone. Within the guttural pouch, the stylopharyngeus muscle can be observed attaching to the ventral aspect of the stylohyoid bone (Fig. 5-3).

The **medial compartment** (Fig. 5-4) is larger than the lateral compartment (Fig. 5-5). The internal carotid artery (ICA) runs from ventral to dorsal in the middle portion of the medial compartment, and forms a sigmoid flexure just before reaching the dorsal limit of the pouch. Cranial nerves IX (glossopharyngeal), X (vagus), XI (accessory) and XII (hypoglossal)

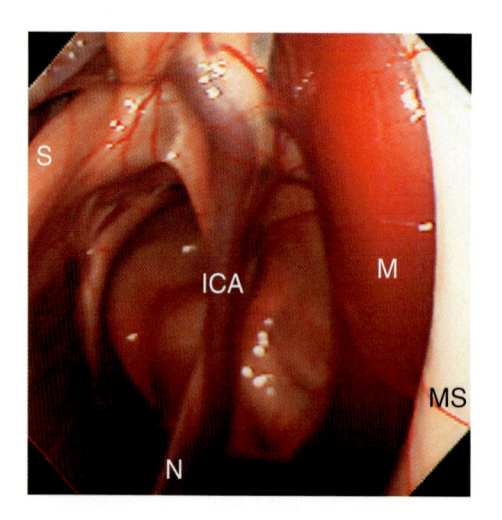

Fig. 5-4: Medial compartment of the right guttural pouch showing stylohyoid bone (S), internal carotid artery (ICA) with its sigmoid flexure dorsally, mucosal fold containing 9th, 10th, 11th and 12th cranial nerves (N), rectus and longus capitus muscles (M) forming the dorso-medial wall of the pouch and median septum (MS) forming the ventro-medial wall of the pouch.

Chapter 5: **Guttural pouches**

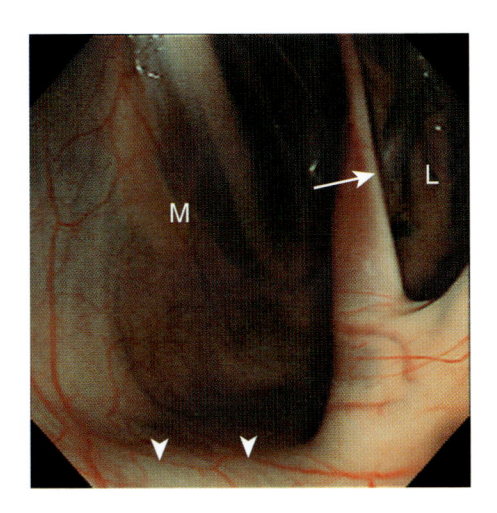

Fig. 5-5: Guttural pouch: photograph taken as the endoscope enters the pouch from the auditory tube. Note the large medial compartment (M) and smaller lateral compartment (L), separated by the stylohoid bone (arrow). Arrowheads point to the floor of the medial compartment which should be examined for evidence of lymphadenopathy or accumulation of abnormal secretions.

emerge from the jugular foramen and hypoglossal canal and course ventrally through the medial compartment of the guttural pouch enveloped in a thin fold of mucosa. These nerves and the sympathetic trunk are intimately associated with the ICA for much of their course within the pouch. The pharyngeal branch of the vagus nerve (X) runs along the floor of the medial compartment before joining the pharyngeal plexus. The floor of the medial compartment (Fig. 5-5) is closely associated with the nasopharynx, which lies ventral to it. The retropharyngeal lymph nodes lie within the tissues separating the nasopharynx and guttural pouch. Lymph nodes are sometimes also apparent in the caudal wall of the medial compartment of the pouch, just lateral and/or medial to the ICA and the mucosal fold containing cranial nerves IX–XII.

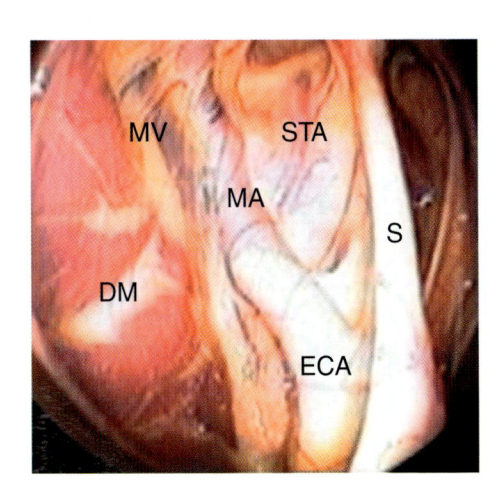

Fig. 5-6: Lateral compartment of the right guttural pouch showing stylohyoid bone (S), external carotid artery (ECA) which continues as the maxillary artery (MA) after giving off a small branch, the superficial temporal artery (STA). The maxillary vein (MV) lies lateral and deep to the maxillary artery. The digastricus muscle (DM) lies on the lateral aspect of the lateral compartment.

Handbook of Equine Respiratory Endoscopy

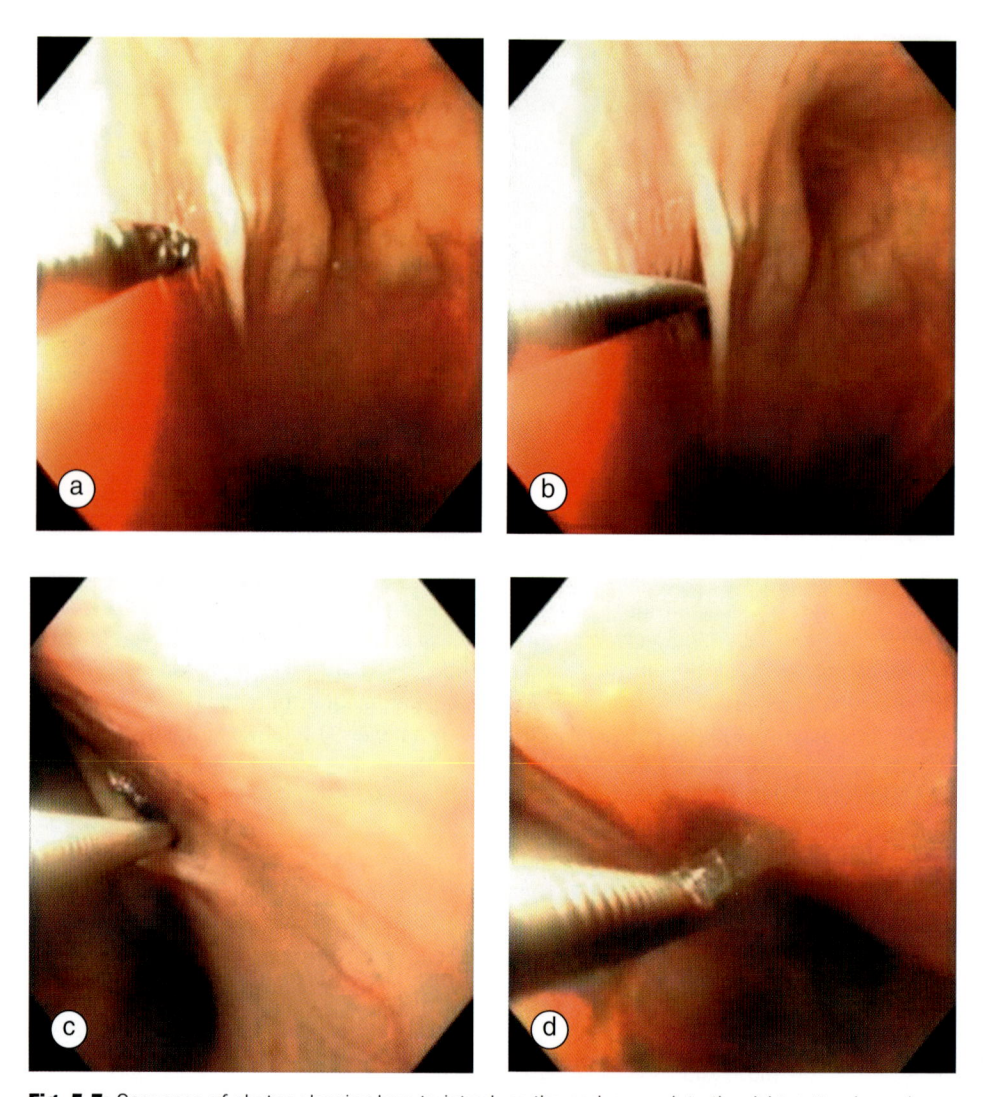

Fig. 5-7: Sequence of photos showing how to introduce the endoscope into the right guttural pouch:
- **a)** The endoscope is passed up the ipsilateral ventral meatus, and positioned just rostral to the ostium of the right guttural pouch in the nasopharynx. Metal biopsy forceps (with the jaws closed) are passed through the biopsy channel of the endoscope.
- **b)** The end of the forceps is pushed caudally through the dorsal part of the guttural pouch ostium for approximately 8 cm and acts as a 'guide' for the endoscope to follow. Care should be taken not to insert an excessive length of probe into the auditory tube, as there is a risk of damaging structures inside the pouch.
- **c)** The endoscope is then rotated, so that the forceps are now positioned as axially as possible with respect to the rest of the endoscope tip, and can be used to elevate the fibrocartilage flap of the ostium, allowing the endoscope to pass into the auditory tube without getting caught on the flap. The endoscope is advanced towards the ostium.
- **d)** The endoscope has entered the auditory tube and is being advanced towards the guttural pouch, still using the biopsy instrument as a guide.

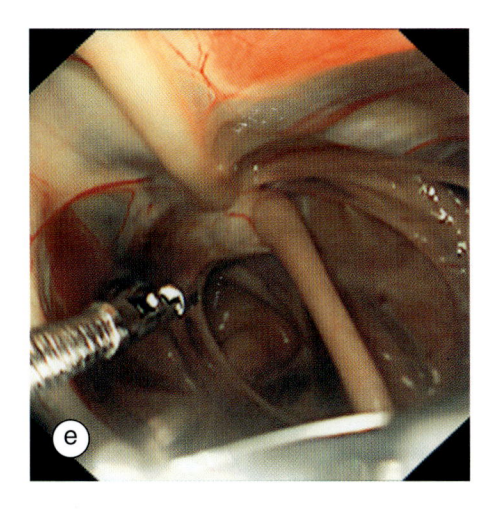

Chapter 5: **Guttural pouches**

Fig. 5-7: *continued*
e) As the tip of the endoscope enters the guttural pouch, the endoscope is rotated back through 180° to view the image the correct way up, and the metal biopsy forceps are promptly withdrawn.

The **lateral compartment** of the guttural pouch (Fig. 5-6) contains the external carotid artery, which enters the pouch ventrally and runs dorsally. The external carotid gives off a small medially directed branch, the superficial temporal artery, and then continues dorsally as the maxillary artery. The maxillary vein runs lateral and deep to the maxillary artery. The digastricus muscle forms part of the lateral wall of the lateral compartment of the guttural pouch.

Tips for endoscopic examination

Endoscopic examination of the guttural pouches requires a small diameter (e.g. <8 mm) endoscope, because the auditory tube is a narrow structure. In addition to the endoscope, some type of probe (e.g. guttural pouch probe [Mila International] or closed transendoscopic biopsy forceps) is required to elevate the fibrocartilaginous ostium of the guttural pouch within the nasopharynx, and guide the endoscope into the auditory tube. Many horses require sedation for safe endoscopic examination of the guttural pouches; should the horse move suddenly whilst the endoscope is in the pouch, the delicate structures contained therein could be damaged. The endoscope should be passed up the ipsilateral ventral meatus until the tip of the endoscope is positioned in the nasopharynx, just rostral to the guttural pouch ostium. Passing the endoscope up the middle meatus may make it more difficult to guide the endoscope into the auditory tube.

A step-by-step description of how to enter the auditory tube and guttural pouch with the endoscope is shown in Fig. 5-7. To enter one guttural pouch, the endoscope has to be rotated through 180° (as shown in Fig. 5-7), due to the eccentric positioning of the biopsy channel in the tip of the endoscope (Fig. 1-3). Rotation positions the probe as far axially as possible with respect to the rest of the endoscope, and ensures that the tip of the endoscope does not get caught on the cartilaginous flap of the ostium when it is advanced towards the auditory tube. On the contralateral side, the eccentric position of the biopsy channel means that the probe is already axially positioned when the endoscope is orientated the correct way up, and rotation is unnecessary.

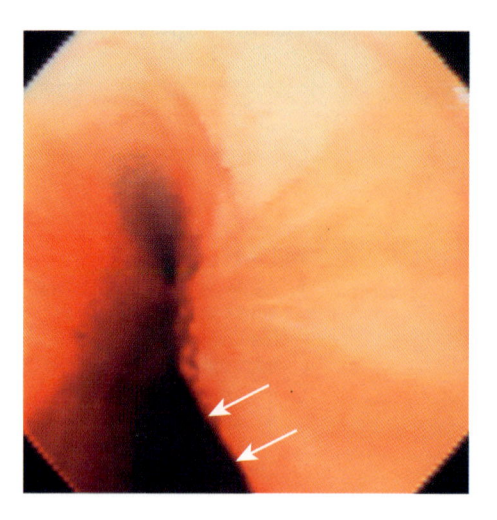

Fig. 5-8: Auditory tube, showing the plica salphingopharyngea (arrows).

The auditory tube is widest at its nasopharyngeal aspect. As the tube continues caudally, the presence of a transverse fold of tissue positioned on its floor (the plica salphingopharyngea) causes it to narrow (Fig. 5-8). The auditory tube enters the guttural pouch approximately one-third of the way up the pouch; this means that fluid accumulates in the ventral parts of the pouch and is only drained when the horse's head is at ground level (e.g. when it is feeding). Swallowing also facilitates drainage.

The medial and lateral compartments of the guttural pouch and the structures within them should be carefully evaluated once the endoscope has entered the pouch. The floor of the medial compartment should be examined for accumulations of fluid or inspissated exudate, blood, or chondroids (Fig. 5-5). The retropharyngeal lymph nodes lie directly beneath the floor of the medial compartment, and if enlarged because of inflammation, infection or neoplasia, they become apparent endoscopically.

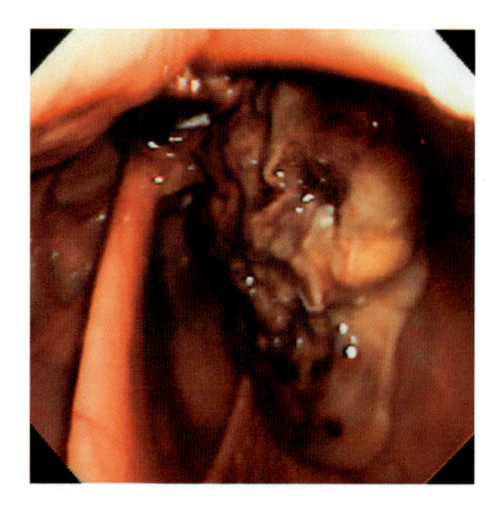

Fig. 5-9: Mycotic guttural pouch infection with *Aspergillus fumigatus*. The fungal plaque is positioned in the dorsal aspect of the medial compartment – it has a predilection site here, at or just below the sigmoid flexure of the internal carotid artery.

Chapter 5: **Guttural pouches**

Abnormalities

Guttural pouch mycosis (GPM)

Aspergillus fumigatus, an opportunistic respiratory pathogen, is responsible for mycotic infection of the guttural pouch. The fungus has a predilection site in the dorsal aspect of the medial compartment of the pouch, usually at or just below the sigmoid flexure of the internal carotid artery (ICA) (Fig. 5-9). The fungus often erodes the major blood vessels that lie within the pouch, and moderate or massive arterial epistaxis unassociated with exercise is a common presenting sign. The fungal plaque often has large amounts of fibrinous material associated with it. Less commonly, the external carotid or maxillary arteries in the lateral compartment may be eroded by the fungal plaque. Although the mycotic infection in GPM is usually unilateral, epistaxis may be unilateral or bilateral, depending on the volume of hemorrhage draining into the nasopharynx, or if mycotic infection has caused erosion of the median septum of the guttural pouch (Fig. 5-10). Occasionally, fungal erosion of the stylohyoid bone may result in stylohyoid osteopathy and/or pathological fracture; affected horses are often dysphagic.

Horses affected with GPM may also show neurological signs due to damage to the cranial nerves and the cranial sympathetic trunk that run within the guttural pouch. These may include pharyngeal dysfunction resulting in dysphagia (Fig. 4-9) (IX, X and XI) with nasal return of saliva/food/water, recurrent laryngeal neuropathy (recurrent laryngeal branch of X), Horner's syndrome (cranial sympathetic nerve) and persistent dorsal displacement of the

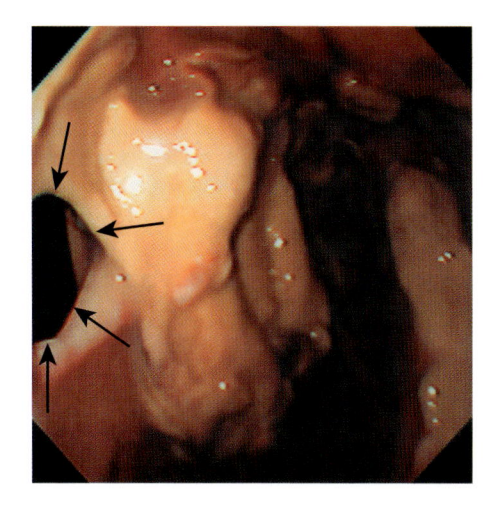

Fig. 5-10: Case of guttural pouch mycosis of the left pouch where the fungal plaque has eroded the thin median septum. A communication is now present into the right pouch (arrows).

soft palate (pharyngeal branch of X). Other clinical signs of guttural pouch mycosis include mucopurulent nasal discharge, swelling of the ipsilateral submandibular lymph nodes and parotid region, hyperextension of the head and neck, and dyspnea.

Endoscopic examination of the nasopharynx may reveal blood, blood clots (Fig. 5-11a) or mucopurulent discharge emanating from the ostium of the affected pouch. If the horse has experienced a recent hemorrhage, great care should be taken when advancing the endoscope into the affected pouch to avoid disturbing the blood clot (Fig. 5-11c), which

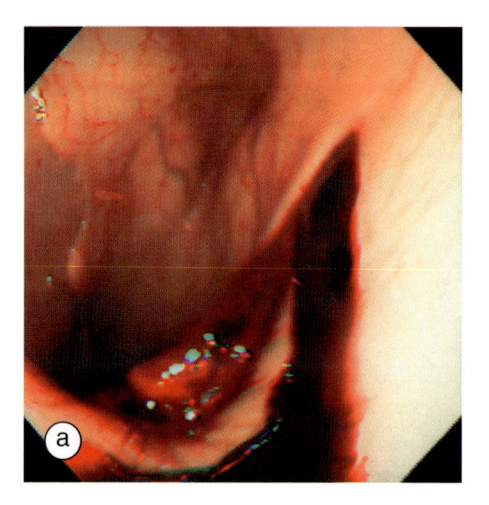

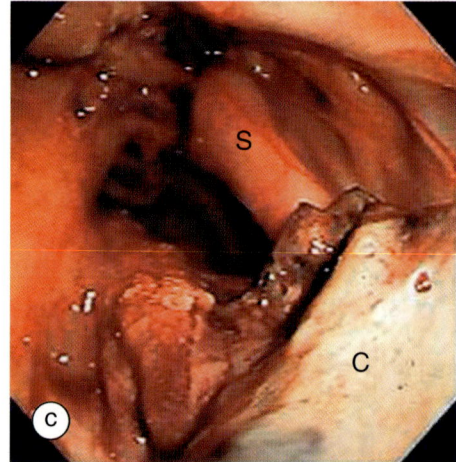

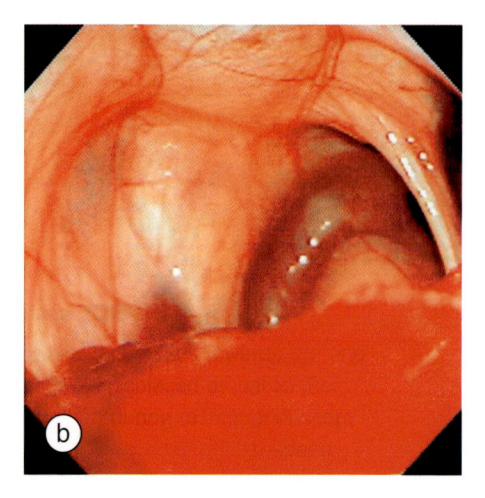

Fig. 5-11: Guttural pouch mycosis.
a) Nasopharynx of a horse with guttural pouch mycosis which has had a recent episode of hemorrhage from the left pouch. There is a large blood clot emanating from the left guttural pouch ostium.
b) Guttural pouch of the same horse, filled with blood.
c) Guttural pouch of the same horse 24 hours after the episode of epistaxis, showing a large blood clot (C) still filling most of the guttural pouch lumen. Dorsal aspect of stylohyoid bone (S).

Chapter 5: **Guttural pouches**

may be sealing the defect in the arterial wall, as this can result in another, possibly fatal, hemorrhage. The history of profuse epistaxis not associated with exercise or trauma plus the endoscopic finding of blood emanating from a guttural pouch ostium provides the clinician with enough evidence to warrant referral to a surgical facility without performing endoscopy of the pouch itself.

Once the horse is in a hospital facility where the affected artery can be surgically occluded, the pouches should be examined endoscopically pre-operatively in order to confirm that GPM is indeed the cause of epistaxis, to verify which pouch is affected (erosion of the median septum may result in blood emanating from the contralateral ostium in the nasopharynx) and to ascertain which artery within the pouch is involved. Determination of the affected artery may not be possible, however, if the affected pouch is still filled with blood (Fig. 5-11b & c).

There is a 50% mortality rate if GPM is left untreated. Treatment of GPM involves surgical occlusion of the affected artery. The efficacy of topical antifungal therapy is controversial because mycotic lesions often resolve after arterial occlusion alone. Topical application of an effective antifungal agent such as natamycin, enilconazole or nystatin solution sprayed via a transendoscopic delivery catheter may help destroy the infective fungus, preventing further damage to nerves and vessels. The physical process of irrigation may additionally assist to break down and eliminate the fungal plaque.

Guttural pouch empyema

Guttural pouch empyema is commonly associated with infection with *Streptococcus equi var. equi* (strangles). Abscesses form in the retropharyngeal lymph nodes (in the floor of the pouch; Fig. 5-12), which then rupture and drain into the lumen of the pouch. Purulent exudate may be seen draining from the guttural pouch ostium into the nasopharynx (Fig. 4-11) and enlarged lymph nodes, liquid exudate or chondroids (Fig. 5-13) may be seen on the floor of the medial compartment of the pouch. Observation of a fluid line within the pouch(es) of a lateral radiograph may help to confirm the diagnosis.

Guttural pouch lavage (Fig. 5-14) or aspiration of fluid which pools in the floor of the medial compartment is easily performed, and bacteriological culture or polymerase chain reaction (PCR) testing of the fluid should confirm the diagnosis of strangles. Chronic carriers of strangles may harbor the bacterium within the guttural pouches without obvious lymphadenopathy being apparent. Horses afflicted with other bacterial (e.g. *Streptococcus zooepidemicus*) or viral upper respiratory tract infections can also occasionally have catarrhal inflammation of the guttural pouch mucosa, which may result in empyema. Horses with chronic catarrhal inflammation of the guttural pouches may occasionally present with neurological signs associated with an extension of the inflammatory process from the mucosa to the cranial nerves located within the walls of the guttural pouch.

Repeated lavage of empyemic guttural pouches using an indwelling Foley catheter or coiled polyurethane guttural pouch catheter (Mila International) may be useful to encourage drainage of purulent material. Horses with retropharyngeal abscessation are most commonly treated with supportive therapy, but a modified Whitehouse approach can be used to

Handbook of Equine Respiratory Endoscopy

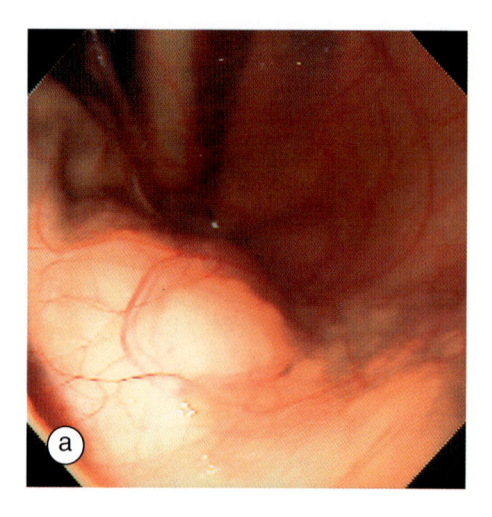

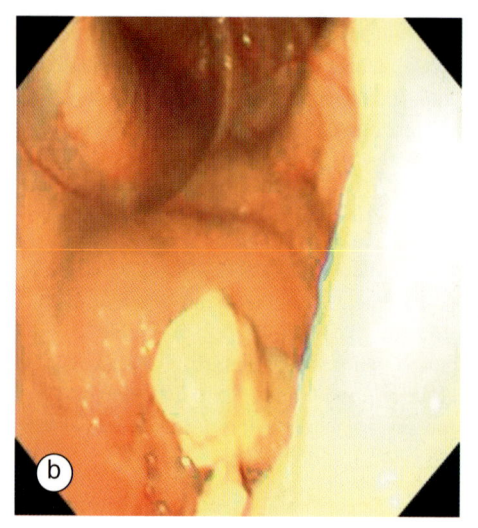

Fig. 5-12a, b: Retropharyngeal lymphadenopathy evident in the floor of the medial compartment of guttural pouches associated with *Streptococcus equi* infection. In **b)**, the abscessated lymph node has burst, releasing thick purulent material.

surgically drain the abscessated lymph nodes, particularly if they are very enlarged and causing respiratory obstruction. Antimicrobial therapy should be reserved for severe cases and those where lymph nodes are already draining.

Chapter 5: **Guttural pouches**

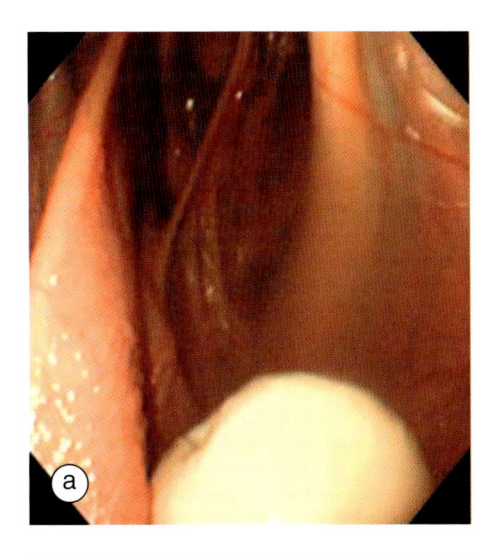

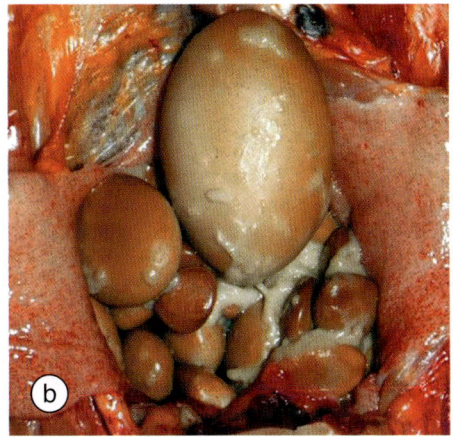

Fig. 5-13: Guttural pouch chondroids.
a) Medial compartment of the guttural pouch of a horse with chronic guttural pouch empyema. A concretion of inspissated purulent material is visible ventrally.
b) Cadaver specimen with multiple large chondroids within the guttural pouch. Photograph courtesy of P. M. Dixon.

Chondroids

Chronic guttural pouch empyema may lead to stagnation of purulent material within the pouch due to impaired mucociliary clearance mechanisms or dysfunction of the drainage ostium. Stagnation leads to inspissation of pus which may subsequently result in chondroid formation (Fig. 5-13).

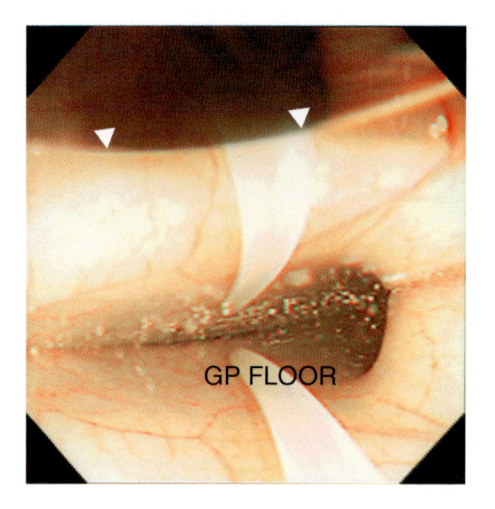

Fig. 5-14: Guttural pouch lavage: a sterile guarded plastic catheter has been introduced via the biopsy channel of the scope, and 10 ml of sterile physiological saline has been injected through this to lavage the guttural pouch. The catheter tip is then directed ventrally into the fluid (top of the fluid is denoted by arrowheads) which accumulates in the ventral aspect of the medial compartment (GP floor) and the fluid aspirated and sent for bacterial culture and/or PCR. This method is used commonly for cases of guttural pouch empyema where infection with *S. equi var. equi* is suspected.

Small chondroids can be removed via the auditory tube using transendoscopic basket forceps (Fig. 5-15), but larger ones must be removed surgically (e.g. using the Whitehouse or modified Whitehouse approach; Fig. 5-16). Alternatively, chondroids can sometimes be reduced into small pieces using a trans-endoscopic snare or by infusion of acetylcysteine into the pouch. The small pieces may then be lavaged from the pouch.

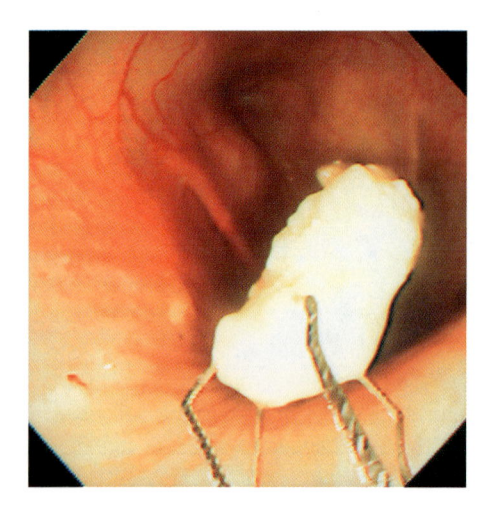

Fig. 5-15: Small guttural pouch chondroid which has been removed from the guttural pouch using transendoscopic basket forceps.

Chapter 5: **Guttural pouches**

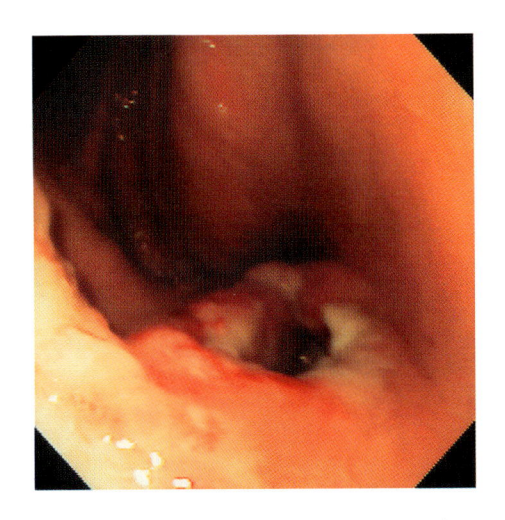

Fig. 5-16: Floor of the medial compartment of the right guttural pouch in a horse which had several chondroids removed surgically using a modified Whitehouse approach. The wound is considered to be contaminated and is therefore left to heal by secondary intention.

Guttural pouch tympany

Guttural pouch tympany is a disorder characterized by excessive amounts of air accumulating within the guttural pouch. The disorder occurs predominantly in young fillies, although it is seen occasionally as an acquired disorder in adult horses. Affected horses have some structural or functional disorder of the auditory tube or the nasopharyngeal ostium, which allows air to enter, but not exit the guttural pouch (i.e. the tube/ostium acts as a one-way valve). Secondary empyema caused by lack of normal drainage of fluid from the pouch frequently occurs concurrently. Clinical signs include a large tympanitic swelling caudal and caudo-ventral to the mandible (Fig. 5-17). Ventral distension of the pouch may cause compression of the roof of the nasopharynx, and hence severely affected animals

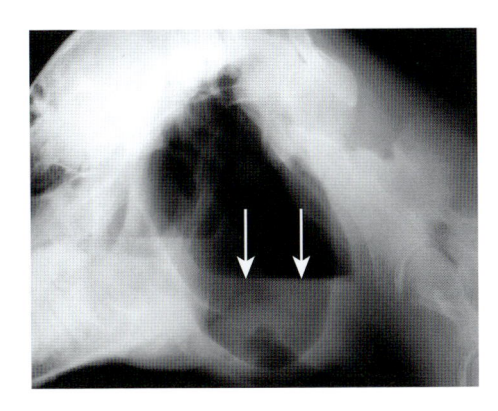

Fig. 5-17: Bilateral guttural pouch tympany: lateral radiograph of 11-day-old filly foal. The guttural pouches are massively distended with air (large radiolucent areas ventral to the base of the skull and the 1st and 2nd cervical vertebrae). Secondary empyema is also present which is radiographically apparent as a horizontal fluid line (arrows) in the ventral part of the pouch. Photograph courtesy of H. McAllister.

may exhibit dysphagia and dyspnea. The median septum separating the pouches is thin, and therefore endoscopic examination of the contralateral pouch may reveal 'bulging' of the septum abaxially into the ventro-medial aspect of the contralateral pouch.

Treatment options include surgical creation of a fistula in the septum that separates the affected and non-affected pouches, so that air can move freely from the affected pouch into the nasopharynx via the contralateral auditory tube. Alternatively, the affected auditory tube and pharyngeal ostium can be enlarged permanently by implanting a Foley catheter into the guttural pouch for several weeks, or for bilateral cases, a fistula can be surgically created between the pouches and the nasopharynx.

Neoplasia

Small melanomas are commonly seen in the guttural pouches of gray horses, often situated in the lateral compartment, on or near the ECA or maxillary artery (Fig. 5-18). These are usually very slow-growing, and hence rarely cause clinical signs. Malignant neoplasms of the guttural pouches are rare, but lymphosarcomas and malignant melanomas are the most frequently observed. Hemangiosarcomas, fibromas and squamous cell carcinomas of the guttural pouch have also been reported. Clinical signs caused by neoplasia of the guttural pouch generally relate to invasion of, or metastasis to, the retropharyngeal lymph nodes, which enlarge, resulting in collapse of the dorsal roof of the nasopharynx, which in turn results in dyspnea and dysphagia (Fig. 4-10).

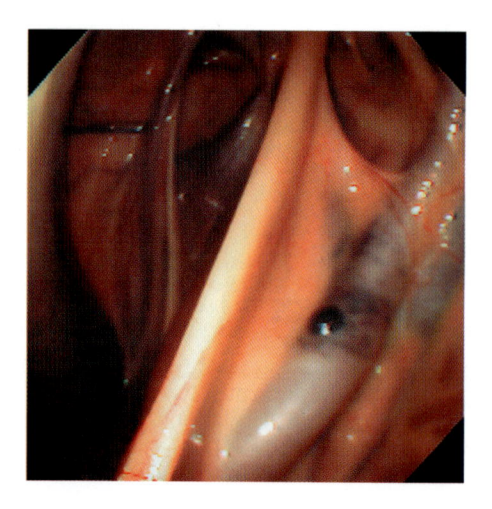

Fig. 5-18: Guttural pouch melanoma. Left guttural pouch of a gray 7-year-old mare, with a small area of melanosis on the ECA in the lateral compartment of the left guttural pouch. This was an incidental finding.

Chapter 5: **Guttural pouches**

Temporohyoid osteopathy

Temporohyoid osteoarthropathy is thought to be a result of primary degenerative joint disease or extension of infection from the middle ear. The dorsal aspect of the stylohyoid bone and squamous portion of the temporal bone become thickened and eventually fuse, predisposing the horse to fracture of the petrous temporal bone and neurological deficits caused by damage to the cranial nerves that exit the skull close to this area. Early clinical signs may be related to irritation of the affected area and include head-shaking and ear-rubbing, but fracture of the petrous temporal bone often causes an acute onset of severe clinical signs. Damage to the vestibulotrochlear nerve (VIII) results in ataxia, head tilt and spontaneous nystagmus. The facial nerve (VII) is also often damaged, resulting in facial paralysis. Affected horses commonly develop corneal ulcers secondary to kerato-conjunctivitis sicca caused by damage to the parasympathetic innervation to the lacrimal gland.

Endoscopy of the affected guttural pouch reveals remodeling of the dorsal aspect of the stylohyoid bone (Fig. 5-19), and sometimes fracture of the body of the stylohyoid bone. Radiographic and/or scintigraphic examination of the skull confirms the diagnosis. Treatment involves administration of systemic antibiotics and non-steroidal anti-inflammatory drugs. Partial ostectomy of the stylohyoid or disarticulation of the hyoid apparatus distally can be performed in horses whose temporohyoid articulation is fused, thus preventing fractures of the temporal bone and hence damage to the cranial nerves.

Rupture of the rectus capitus and longus capitus muscles

The longus capitis and rectus capitis ventralis muscles are flexor muscles of the head. They originate from the cranial cervical vertebrae, and insert onto the basilar portion of the occipital bone and the body of the basisphenoid bone. A portion of these muscles is visible endoscopically in the dorso-medial aspect of the medial compartment (Fig. 5-4). The longus capitis or rectus capitis ventralis muscles may rupture or become avulsed from the basisphenoid or occipital bones when a horse rears and falls over backwards, and the

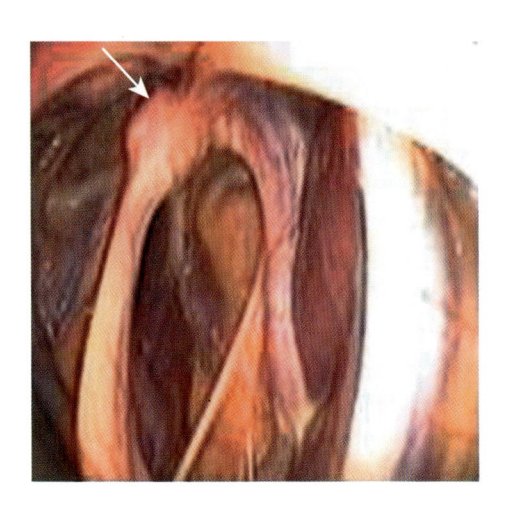

Fig. 5-19: Temporohyoid osteopathy. Note the remodeling of the dorso-lateral aspect of the stylohyoid bone within the right guttural pouch, with marked bony proliferation present. Endoscopy of the guttural pouch is a very sensitive diagnostic tool for this disorder.

damaged muscles may hemorrhage into the guttural pouch. Epistaxis and neurological signs caused by intracranial trauma occur commonly with this injury.

A large hematoma forms within the guttural pouches, which may cause the pharyngeal roof to deviate ventrally. Affected horses may also have a painful external swelling of the retropharyngeal area. Endoscopically, blood clots or fresh blood may be seen emanating from one or both ostia of the guttural pouches, and therefore this condition must be differentiated from GPM by endoscopic examination of the affected pouch. A lateral radiograph of the base of the skull may show avulsed bone fragments that originate from the ventral part of the basisphenoid bone. In the absence of neurological signs, conservative treatment may be successful, but horses with neurological signs usually have a very poor prognosis for recovery.

FURTHER READING

Blazyczek I, Hamann H, Deegen E, Distl O, Ohnesorge B 2004 Retrospective analysis of 50 cases of guttural pouch tympany in foals. Veterinary Record 154:261–2

Edwards B and Greet T 2006 Disorders of the Guttural Pouch. In: Equine Respiratory Medicine and Surgery. Eds: McGorum, Robinson Schumacher and Dixon. Saunders

Judy CE, Chaffin MK, Cohen ND 1999 Empyema of the guttural pouch (auditory tube diverticulum) in horses: 91 cases (1977–1997). Journal of the American Veterinary Medical Association 215:1666–70

Sweeney CR, Freeman DE, Sweeney RW et al. 1993 Hemorrhage into the guttural pouch (auditory tube diverticulum) associated with rupture of the longus capitis muscle in three horses. Journal of the American Veterinary Medical Association 202:1129–31

Walker AM, Sellon DC, Cornelisse CJ et al. Temporohyoid osteoarthropathy in 33 horses (1993–2000). Journal of Veterinary Internal Medicine 16:697–703

Chapter preview

Normal anatomy 67

Tips for endoscopic examination 69

Abnormalities 69
    Recurrent laryngeal neuropathy (RLN) 69
    Arytenoid chondritis 74
    Idiopathic mucosal defects of the arytenoid cartilages 76
    Fourth branchial arch defects (4-BAD, cricopharyngeal-laryngeal dysplasia) 77
    Axial deviation of the aryepiglottic folds 79
    Epiglottic entrapment 80
    Subepiglottic cysts 83
    Epiglottitis 84
    Epiglottic hypoplasia/flaccidity 84
    Subepiglottic ulceration 86

Further reading 87

6: Larynx

Normal anatomy

The equine larynx consists of the epiglottic, paired arytenoid, thyroid and cricoid cartilages (Fig. 6-1). Only the rostral portion of the larynx consisting of the epiglottis and the paired corniculate processes of the arytenoid cartilages can be easily viewed endoscopically (Fig. 6-2). The epiglottic cartilage is leaf-shaped and ventrally curved, has prominent blood vessels visible on its pharyngeal surface and serrated lateral margins. It is connected to the lateral aspect of the arytenoid cartilages by the fleshy aryepiglottic folds which attach to its caudo-lateral margins. The aryepiglottic folds are continuous with the subepiglottic mucosal folds (glossoepiglottic folds) which cover the hyoepiglotticus muscles and ligaments, and extend ventrally to the base of the tongue. The paired corniculate processes of the arytenoid cartilages form the dorsal border of the rima glottidis and have a wide range of movement;

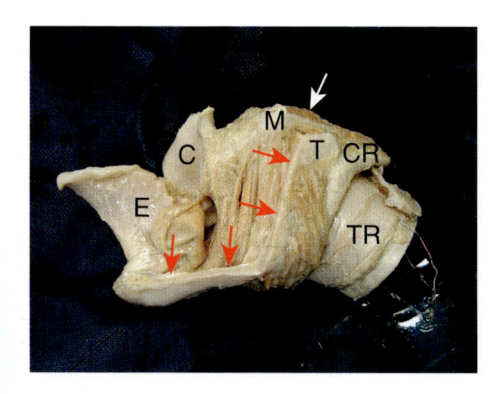

Fig. 6-1: Cadaver larynx – lateral aspect with rostral part of the thyroid cartilage removed (red arrows). E = epiglottis, C = corniculate process of the left arytenoid cartilage, M = muscular process of the left arytenoid cartilage, T = thyroid cartilage, CR = cricoid cartilage and TR = trachea. The crico-arytenoideus dorsalis muscle (white arrow) runs on the dorsal aspect of the larynx between the cricoid cartilage and the muscular process of the arytenoid cartilage.

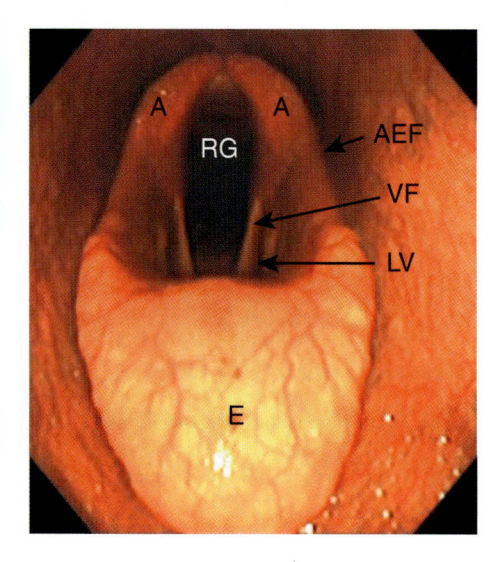

Fig. 6-2: Normal larynx during quiet breathing. The epiglottic cartilage (E) has prominent blood vessels, serrated edges and a ventral 'leaf-shaped' curvature. The paired corniculate processes of the arytenoid cartilages (A) form the dorsal border of the rima glottidis (RG). They are connected to the epiglottis by the aryepiglottic folds (AEF), and to the thyroid cartilage by the vocal folds (VF). The laryngeal ventricles (LV) lie abaxial to the vocal folds.

adduction describes movement towards the midline, while abduction describes movement away from the midline.

The vocal folds are normally two taut bands of tissue which form the ventro-lateral borders of the rima glottidis; they extend from the vocal processes on the ventro-medial aspect of each arytenoid to the ventral midline of the thyroid cartilage. The laryngeal ventricles are

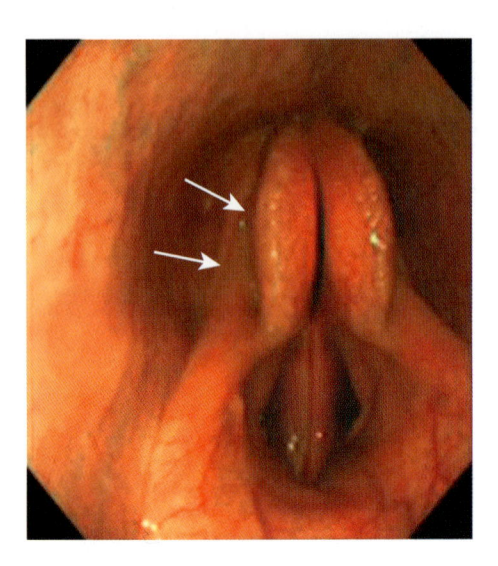

Fig. 6-3: Larynx just prior to swallowing – the arytenoid cartilages are adducted to protect the lower airway from food material, and the entrance to the esophagus can be seen (arrows).

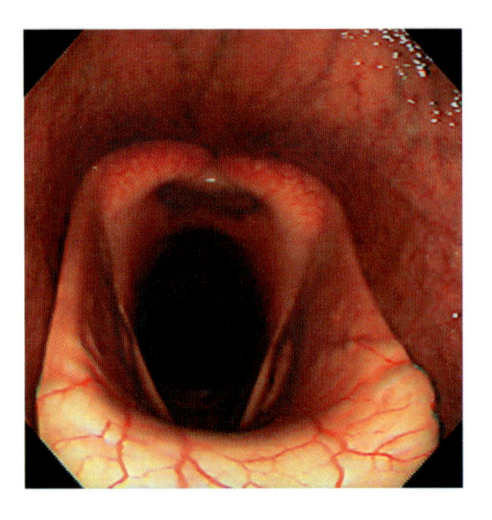

Fig. 6-4: Larynx immediately after swallowing – note the maximal but slightly asymmetrical abduction of the arytenoid cartilages (this horse had grade 3.1 laryngeal function at rest, and grade A laryngeal function at exercise [see Tables 6-1 and 8-1]).

blind-ending mucosal outpouchings, the openings to which are positioned just abaxial and rostral to each vocal fold. The caudal aspect of the larynx is continuous with the trachea and can be viewed by passing the endoscope through the rima glottidis.

The rostral portion of the larynx is a dynamic structure. During exercise the larynx maintains as large an airway as possible by abduction of both arytenoid cartilages. During swallowing, adduction of the arytenoid cartilages and vocal folds (Fig. 6-3) and retroversion of the epiglottis protect the lower airways from aspiration of food material, and immediately after swallowing, full arytenoid abduction occurs (Fig. 6-4).

Tips for endoscopic examination

Sedating a horse can markedly affect the appearance and function of its larynx and should therefore be avoided when performing laryngoscopy. To view a full range of arytenoid movement during endoscopy of the resting horse, the larynx should be observed during quiet breathing, after swallowing (when the arytenoids should abduct maximally) and during nasal occlusion.

Abnormalities such as dorsal displacement of the soft palate and axial deviation of the aryepiglottic folds may be observed during nasal occlusion, but the significance of these findings with respect to how the larynx functions when the horse exercises is questionable.

To achieve consistency when assessing the endoscopic appearance of the larynx, the same nostril should be used routinely for insertion of the endoscope (the author uses the right nostril). Endoscopy at rest, rather than immediately after exercise, allows for observation of a wider range of laryngeal movements because subtleties in laryngeal asymmetry and asynchrony may be more difficult to assess immediately post exercise due to hyperventilation.

Abnormalities

Recurrent laryngeal neuropathy (RLN)

Recurrent laryngeal neuropathy (laryngeal paralysis, idiopathic laryngeal hemiplegia or 'roaring') is the most common cause of equine upper respiratory tract obstruction. It occurs most commonly in tall horses, and becoming increasingly rare in horses less than 15.2hh (1.55m). The vast majority of cases are idiopathic and involve a distal axonopathy of the left recurrent laryngeal nerve. This nerve is the longest nerve in the body and innervates both the principal abductor (crico-arytenoideus dorsalis; Fig. 6-1) and adductor (crico-arytenoideus lateralis) muscles of the left side of the larynx. The most common cause of right-sided laryngeal dysfunction is not RLN, but fourth branchial arch defect. There is evidence to support a degree of heritability of RLN, but the mechanisms and mode of inheritance remain unclear. Occasionally, the recurrent laryngeal nerve can be damaged iatrogenically (most commonly by perivascular injection of irritant drugs), resulting in laryngeal hemiplegia. Other disease processes such as guttural pouch mycosis or cranial thoracic masses may also damage the nerve, resulting in reduced motility of the ipsilateral arytenoid cartilage.

Affected horses often show clinical signs when they are first introduced to work, but the disorder can be progressive and appearance or deterioration of clinical signs can occur over weeks to years at any age. Clinical signs consist of the production of abnormal inspiratory noises at exercise, ranging from a high-pitched 'whistle' to a harsh 'roar', which is often accompanied by exercise intolerance. The abnormal respiratory noises stop very soon after exercise is ceased, and prolonged post-exertional tachypnea is not usually observed in horses with RLN, unless concurrent lower respiratory disease is present.

Diagnosis of RLN is based on a combination of laryngeal palpation for evidence of muscular atrophy, laryngoscopy, and a 'wind' test which allows the veterinarian to hear any abnormal sounds being produced at exercise. High-speed treadmill endoscopy is sometimes indicated to evaluate the function of the larynx during strenuous exercise (see Chapter 8).

Table 6-1: Grading system of laryngeal function performed in the standing unsedated horse

Grade	Description	Subgrade
1	All arytenoid cartilage movements are synchronous and symmetrical and full arytenoid cartilage abduction can be achieved and maintained	
2	Arytenoid cartilage movements are asynchronous and/or larynx is asymmetrical at times but full arytenoid cartilage abduction can be achieved and maintained	.1: Transient asynchrony, flutter or delayed movements are seen
		.2: There is asymmetry of the rima glottidis much of the time due to reduced mobility of the affected arytenoid and vocal fold but there are occasions, typically after swallowing or nasal occlusion when full symmetrical abduction is achieved and maintained
3	Arytenoid cartilage movements are asynchronous and/or asymmetrical. Full arytenoid cartilage abduction cannot be achieved and maintained	.1: There is asymmetry of the rima glottidis much of the time due to reduced mobility of the arytenoid and vocal fold but there are occasions, typically after swallowing or nasal occlusion when full symmetrical abduction is achieved but not maintained
		.2: Obvious arytenoid abductor deficit and arytenoid asymmetry. Full abduction is never achieved
		.3: Marked but not total arytenoid abductor deficit and asymmetry with little arytenoid movement. Full abduction is never achieved
4	Complete immobility of the arytenoid cartilage and vocal fold	

Source: Proceedings of the Havermeyer Foundation Monograph Series No. 11 (Equine Recurrent Laryngeal Neuropathy) 2003, p 96

Chapter 6: Larynx

Obstruction of the airway at exercise is caused by inability to maintain full abduction of the left arytenoid cartilage. This is worse during inspiration, when large negative pressures are generated, causing collapse of the corniculate process and the ipsilateral vocal fold into the airway. An endoscopic grading system for laryngeal function has been established to permit consistency of interpretation between clinicians and this is shown in Table 6-1. Both symmetry of the arytenoids (Figs 6-5, 6-6 and 6-7) and synchrony of their movement must be assessed in order to grade horses accurately. The larynx cannot be graded from a still photograph because the endoscopist is evaluating a dynamic process.

Horses that can achieve and maintain full abduction of the arytenoid cartilages (grades 1 and 2) are unlikely to experience collapse of an arytenoid or vocal fold while exercising. Inability to achieve full abduction of the affected arytenoid cartilage (grades 3.2, 3.3 and 4) is likely to be associated with varying degrees of compromised respiratory function during exercise. There is currently no consensus on the significance of arytenoid abduction that is achieved but not maintained (grade 3.1); such horses may have normal laryngeal function during exercise, or they may experience collapse of the arytenoid cartilage and/or vocal fold.

Endoscopic examination of weanlings for presence of RLN is an unreliable predictor of their laryngeal appearance as yearlings; approximately 20% of foals 'deteriorate' and 20% 'improve' compared with their laryngeal grade as yearlings. Thoroughbred yearlings with grade 1 and 2 laryngeal function have been reported to have significantly better racing performance as adults than yearlings with grade 3 laryngeal function.

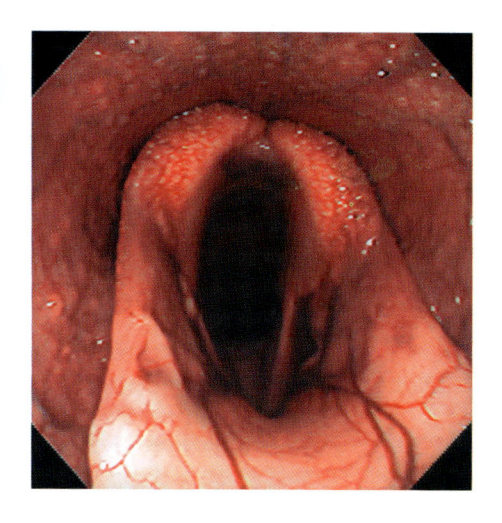

Fig. 6-5: Recurrent laryngeal neuropathy. Grade 2.2 laryngeal function. Photograph taken during quiet breathing – the left arytenoid cartilage is not as fully abducted as the right, therefore there is mild asymmetry of the rima glottidis. After swallowing, this horse was able to achieve and maintain full abduction of the left arytenoid.

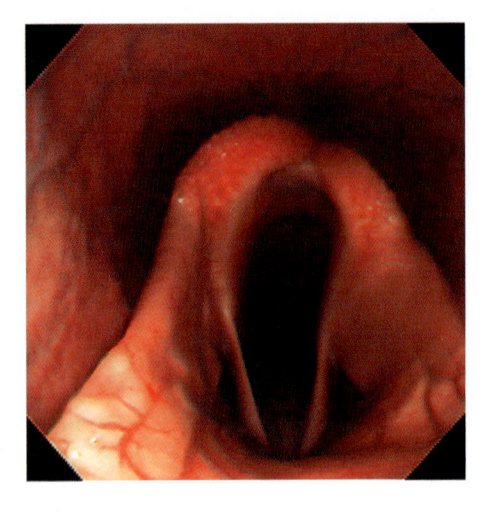

Fig. 6-6: Recurrent laryngeal neuropathy. Grade 3.2 laryngeal function at rest. Photograph taken during quiet breathing – there is obvious asymmetry of the rima glottidis, due to reduced mobility of the left arytenoid cartilage. Full abduction of the left arytenoid was never achieved.

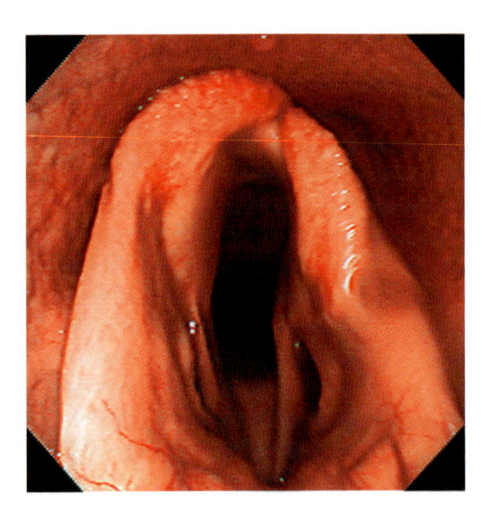

Fig. 6-7: Recurrent laryngeal neuropathy. Grade 4 laryngeal function. Photograph taken during quiet breathing – note how the right arytenoid is abducted, yet the left arytenoid is still hanging in the midline, showing marked asymmetry. This horse had no residual movement of its left arytenoid.

Surgical treatments for RLN include prosthetic laryngoplasty ('tie-back' procedure), ventriculectomy ('Hobday' procedure), vocal cordectomy, neuromuscular pedicle grafts, arytenoidectomy and tracheostomy. Prosthetic laryngoplasty is the most commonly used treatment, and aims to fix the left arytenoid in an abducted position, thereby preventing it from collapsing into the airway during inspiration (Fig. 6-8). Although laryngoplasty can restore normal airflow in horses with complete hemiplegia, the left arytenoid cartilage can no longer adduct to protect the lower airways from inhalation of food during swallowing.

Chapter 6: **Larynx**

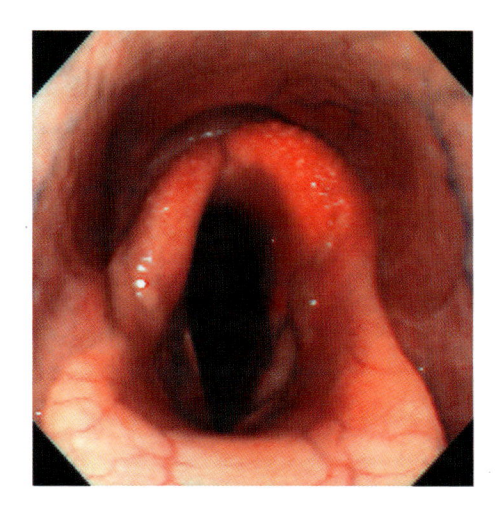

Fig. 6-8: Larynx 6 days after prosthetic laryngoplasty ('tie-back') and ventriculocordectomy procedures for treatment of RLN. Note how the left arytenoid is now fixed in a moderately abducted position.

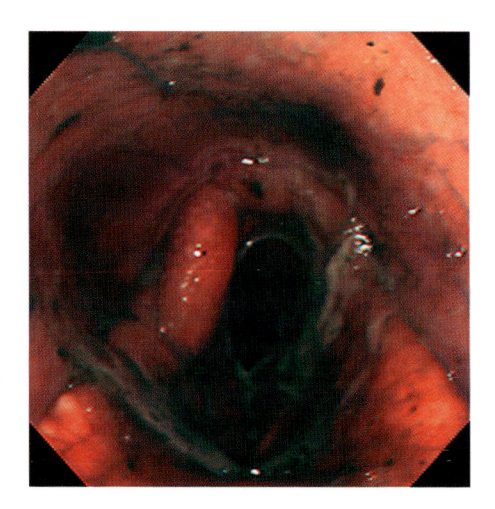

Fig. 6-9: Larynx 1 day after prosthetic laryngoplasty procedure. The left arytenoid is fixed in a hyperabducted position. Food material is present in the pharynx and larynx and is also being aspirated into the trachea. This is a common complication after laryngoplasty. In most cases the dysphagia improves after a few days to weeks; however, a minority of cases will require a second surgery to remove or loosen the prosthesis.

Aspiration of food is therefore a common, but usually short-term complication of this surgery (Fig. 6-9). Ventriculocordectomy (ventriculectomy and vocal cordectomy) can be performed alone (Fig. 6-10) to treat mildly affected horses or horses intended for low-level activities, or in conjunction with laryngoplasty. Ventriculocordectomy is thought to be an important factor in reducing abnormal inspiratory sounds associated with RLN.

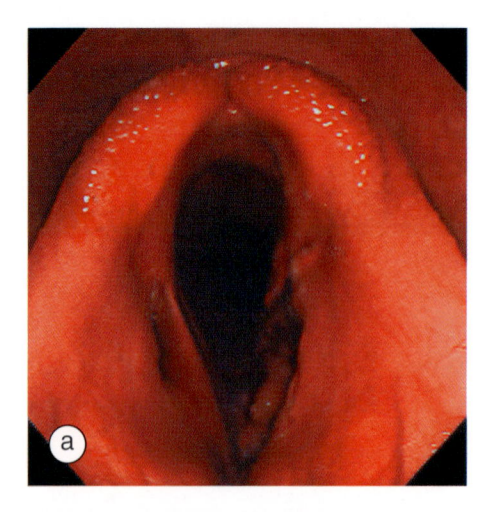

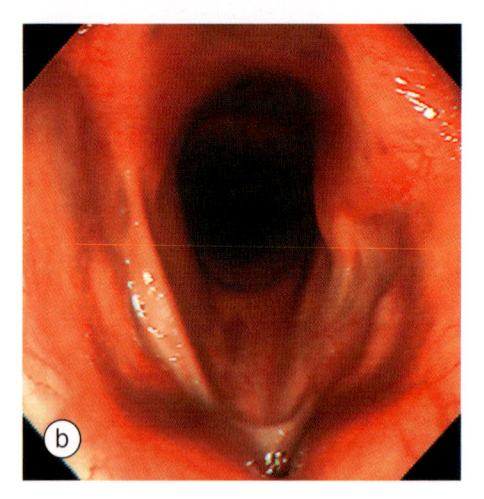

Fig. 6-10: Left-sided vocal cordectomy and bilateral ventriculectomy sites:
a) One day post-operatively.
b) Six weeks post-operatively.

Arytenoid chondritis

Young male Thoroughbreds are particularly predisposed to developing arytenoid chondritis, which is a disorder characterized by infection and inflammation of one or both arytenoid cartilages, but its etiology is currently unclear. The disorder occurs more commonly in the USA than in Europe.

Clinical signs include abnormal respiratory sounds at exercise and reduced athletic performance. Stridor may be heard at rest in severely affected horses. Endoscopically, the affected arytenoid cartilage(s) usually appear thickened, edematous and reddened and may have a distorted outline. They show reduced motility, axial displacement towards the midline, and often have sinus tracts or granulomatous masses on their axial surfaces (Figs 6-11, 6-12), with 'kissing' lesions present on the contralateral arytenoid (Fig. 6-12).

Chapter 6: **Larynx**

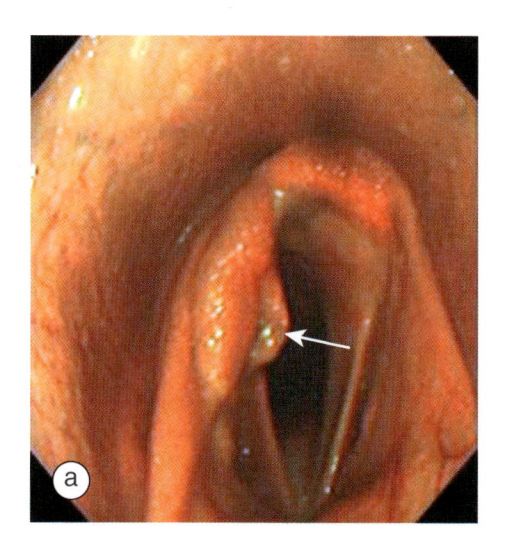

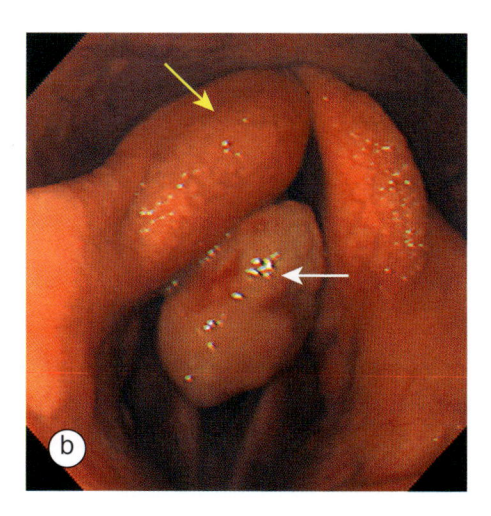

Fig. 6-11: Arytenoid chondritis.
a) Unilateral arytenoid chondritis affecting the right arytenoid cartilage. The affected cartilage is misshapen and has a small granuloma on its axial surface (arrow). This photograph was taken immediately after swallowing, and shows markedly reduced abduction of the right arytenoid compared with the left arytenoid, which is fully abducted.
b) Very large granuloma (white arrow) attached to the right arytenoid which is obstructing the rima glottidis. Note the edematous appearance of the arytenoid cartilage (yellow arrow), and lack of abduction on this side.

The palatopharyngeal arch may be displaced rostrally (RDPA) (Fig. 6-12). Radiographic examination of the affected area may reveal abnormal calcification of affected cartilages, which is associated with a poor prognosis for return to athletic function.

Medical treatment with long-term systemic and topical antibiotics and NSAIDs is rarely successful, and surgical removal of the affected cartilage is usually necessary. Partial (Fig. 6-13), subtotal or total arytenoidectomy techniques have been described. Partial

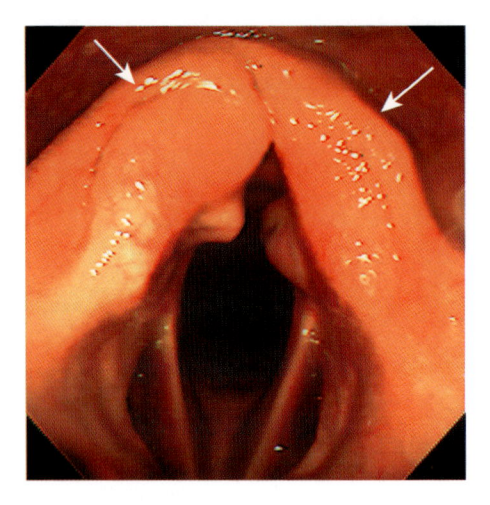

Fig. 6-12: Bilateral arytenoid chondritis. Both arytenoid cartilages are very swollen, edematous and misshapen and exhibit markedly reduced motility. There are granulomas on the axial aspects of both arytenoids. Secondary rostral displacement of the palatopharyngeal arch has also occurred (arrows), forming a 'fold' of soft tissue over the dorsal aspect of the arytenoids.

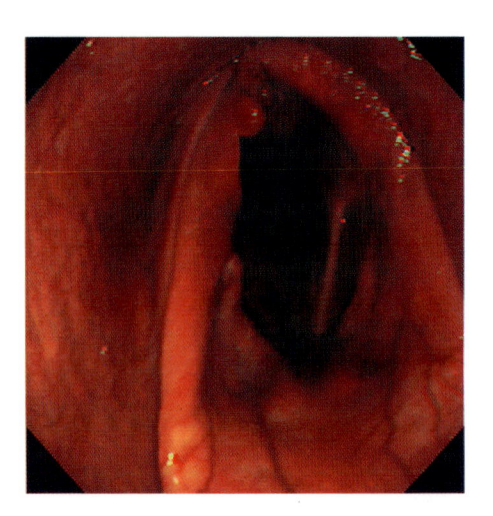

Fig. 6-13: Horse, 4 days after unilateral (right-sided) partial arytenoidectomy.

arytenoidectomy is the best technique for improving respiratory function and is recommended for performance horses. Dyspnea, dysphagia and coughing (particularly associated with eating) are common complications of arytenoidectomy. Granulomatous lesions may be removed using transendoscopic laser surgery, if the underlying cartilage appears grossly normal and has a good range of movement.

Idiopathic mucosal defects of the arytenoid cartilages

Ulceration of the arytenoid cartilage mucosa has been reported to occur in 0.6% of Thoroughbred yearlings. The etiology of these lesions is unknown. Important contributing

Chapter 6: Larynx

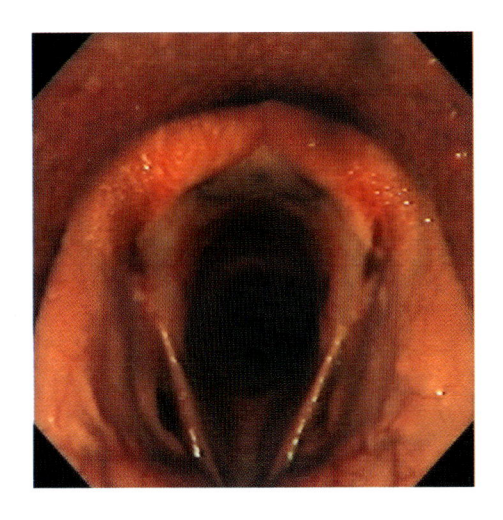

Fig. 6-14: Mucosal erosions on the vocal processes of both arytenoids (just above the attachment of the vocal folds). These lesions may progress to mucosal ulceration.

factors are thought to include an unidentified infectious agent which causes mucosal inflammation at the rostral margin of the vocal processes, and forceful closure of the arytenoid cartilages which may occur during exercise or vocalization. Lesions are usually positioned on the ventral aspect of the arytenoid, just above the dorsal attachment of the vocal cord (Fig. 6-14). The majority of such lesions heal without complications after medical treatment consisting of restricted exercise and systemic and topical antibiotics and NSAIDs. However, occasionally, lesions progress, resulting in development of granulomas or arytenoid chondritis.

Fourth branchial arch defects (4-BAD, cricopharyngeal-laryngeal dysplasia)

Fourth branchial arch syndrome is a congenital disorder, resulting from aplasia or dysplasia of some or all of the derivatives of the embryonic fourth branchial arch. These include the thyroid cartilage, the cricothyroid articulation, the cricopharyngeus muscles (cranial esophageal sphincter) and the cricothyroideus muscles. The right side is affected more commonly than the left, and the condition can also occur bilaterally.

Clinical signs of 4-BAD can be variable, depending on which structures are involved and the severity of the defects. If the thyroid cartilage or the cricothyroid articulation is affected, the action of the crico-arytenoideus dorsalis muscle is diminished, reducing the horse's ability to abduct the arytenoid cartilage. This often leads to abnormal respiratory noise during exercise and poor performance. If the cricopharyngeus muscles are hypoplastic or absent, horses are unable to effectively close the upper esophageal sphincter, resulting in aerophagia which may manifest as chronic eructation or recurrent colic. Other clinical signs observed with this disorder include coughing and nasal discharge.

Palpation of the affected larynx reveals a wide gap between the caudal margin of the thyroid and the rostral edge of the cricoid on one or both sides in most cases; in the normal horse these two structures overlap (Fig. 6-1). Endoscopic examination of the larynx may reveal

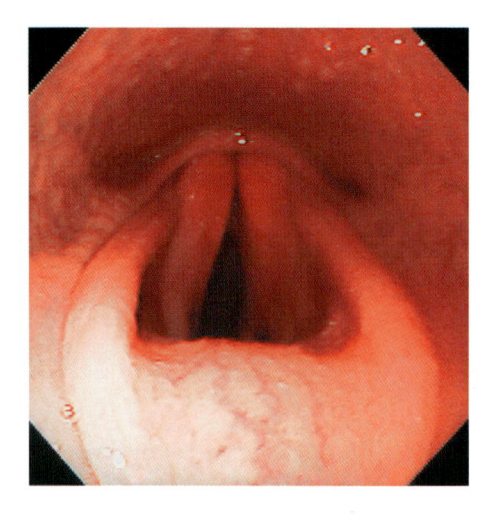

Fig. 6-15: Two-week-old foal with bilateral fourth branchial arch defects. This foal presented with nasal regurgitation of milk. Both arytenoids have reduced motility, being unable to fully abduct, and RDPA is also present, forming a 'cowl' over the dorsal aspect of both arytenoids.

rostral displacement of the palatopharyngeal arch (RDPA), characterized by a cowl of tissue, formed by the caudal pillars of the soft palate, which may partly obscure the dorsal corniculate processes (Fig. 6-15). One or both arytenoids may be unable to fully abduct, mimicking RLN (Figs 6-15 and 6-16). A minority of horses with 4-BAD appear normal during resting endoscopy, but when the horse undergoes high-speed treadmill endoscopy, dynamic RDPA, arytenoid collapse or vocal fold collapse may develop (Fig. 8-13). Lateral radiographs of the laryngeal and cranial cervical region of affected horses will often show an abnormal column of air in the proximal cervical esophagus, and a soft tissue opacity ('dew drop') intruding into this air column, dorsal and rostral to the arytenoid cartilages, which represents RDPA (Fig. 6-17). It should be noted that RDPA and aerophagia may occur in normal horses that have been sedated and therefore endoscopy and radiography of horses suspected of being afflicted with 4-BAD must be performed without chemical restraint.

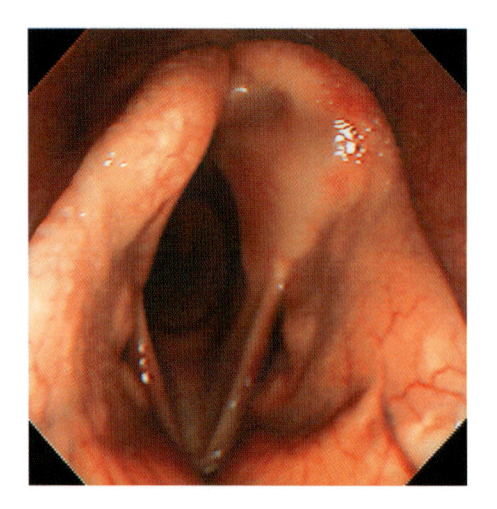

Fig. 6-16: Right-sided fourth branchial arch defects. Endoscopy of the larynx showed sluggish motility of the right arytenoid cartilage, which is only partially abducted (compared with the left arytenoid) in this photograph.

Chapter 6: **Larynx**

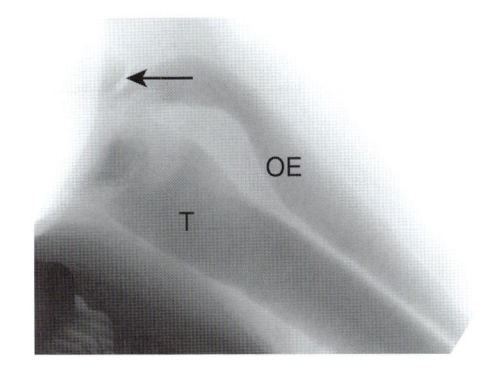

Fig. 6-17: Lateral radiograph of unsedated horse with fourth branchial arch defects. Note the abnormal amount of air within the esophageal lumen (OE). There is a soft tissue density 'dew drop' (arrow) that impinges into this column of air dorsal to the rostral part of the larynx caused by the RDPA. T = Tracheal lumen.

There is no effective treatment for horses affected with 4-BAD, and attempts at surgical correction are usually unsuccessful. Affected horses usually cannot compete in strenuous pursuits such as racing, but are often capable of performing less arduous work. Tracheostomy may provide a means of bypassing the site of airway obstruction and establishing airway efficiency; however, the results are not considered to be aesthetically acceptable by many owners.

Axial deviation of the aryepiglottic folds (Fig. 6-18)

This disorder usually only occurs at fast exercise, but it may occasionally be seen during resting endoscopy when the nostrils are temporarily occluded. The significance of this finding in the resting horse is not known. This disorder is covered in more detail in Chapter 8.

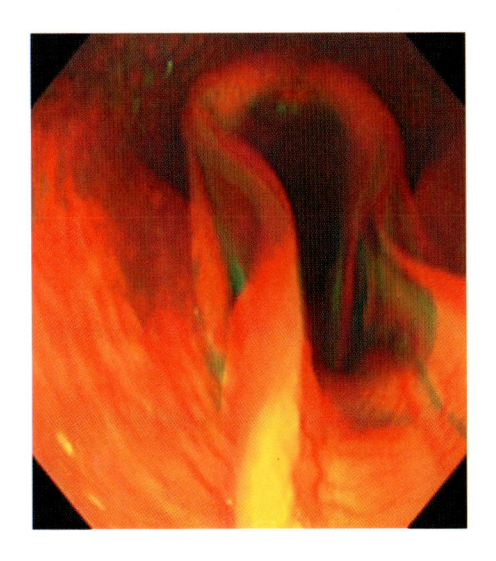

Fig. 6-18: Moderate bilateral axial deviation of the aryepiglottic folds which is occurring at fast exercise (photograph taken during high-speed treadmill endoscopy).

Epiglottic entrapment

Epiglottic entrapment occurs when the epiglottic cartilage becomes entrapped within the subepiglottic (glossoepiglottic) and aryepiglottic mucosal folds. Epiglottic hypoplasia predisposes horses to this disorder, but epiglottic entrapment is also frequently seen in horses with normal epiglottic size and appearance. Horses with epiglottic entrapment may be asymptomatic or demonstrate a range of clinical signs. During fast work, affected horses may make a vibrant expiratory noise or both inspiratory and expiratory noises or no abnormal noise at all. In some cases, epiglottal entrapment does not appear to impair ventilation, even at maximal exercise and this may be related to individual variation in the tightness of the entrapping fold of mucosa. Occasionally, epiglottic entrapment may occur intermittently or only during exercise (see Chapter 8).

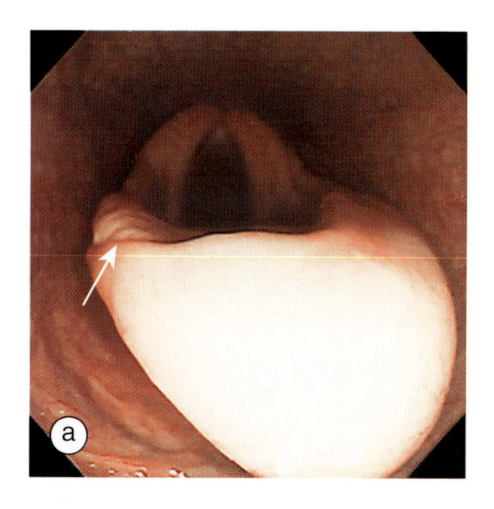

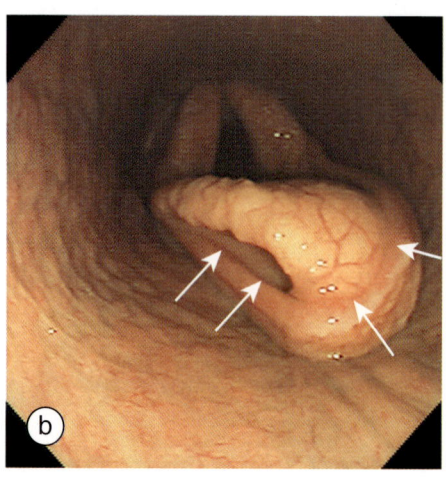

Fig. 6-19: Epiglottal entrapment. The epiglottis has become trapped in the glossoepiglottal and aryepiglottic folds. **a)** The prominent blood vessels on the epiglottal surface and its serrated lateral margins are no longer visible. An arrow points to the edge of the entrapping fold. **b)** The epiglottis is only partially entrapped. Arrows point to the edges of the entrapping fold.

Chapter 6: **Larynx**

Abnormalities seen during endoscopic examination of affected horses include loss of the normal prominent vasculature and serrated lateral margins of the epiglottis, which are replaced by the smooth mucosa of the entrapping membrane (Fig. 6-19). If the entrapment is chronic, inflammation and ulceration of the entrapping fold of mucosa is common (Fig. 6-20). The entrapping fold can be resected via a laryngotomy incision, or axially divided using transendoscopic laser surgery (Fig. 6-21) or a hooked bistoury passed *per nasum* (Fig. 6-22) or *per os*.

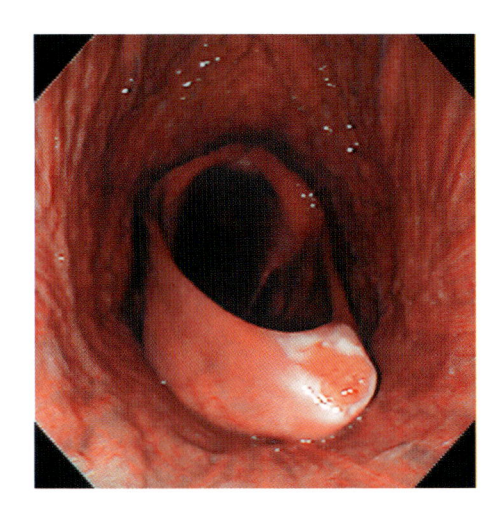

Fig. 6-20: Chronic epiglottal entrapment with ulceration of the entrapping mucosa.

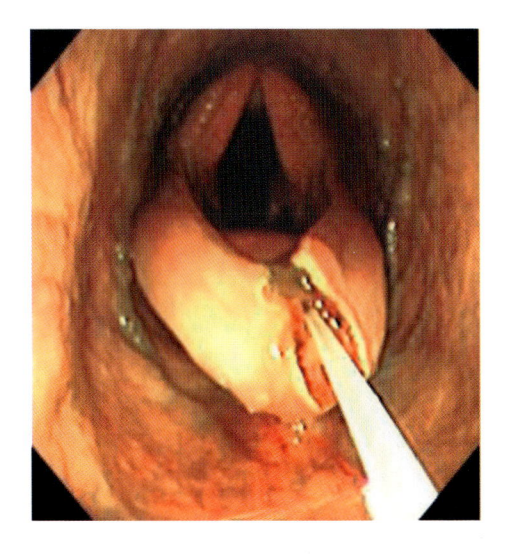

Fig. 6-21: Horse with entrapped epiglottis undergoing axial sectioning with a transendoscopic diode laser; a partial thickness cut has been made using the laser, which is then deepened until the epiglottic cartilage becomes visible.

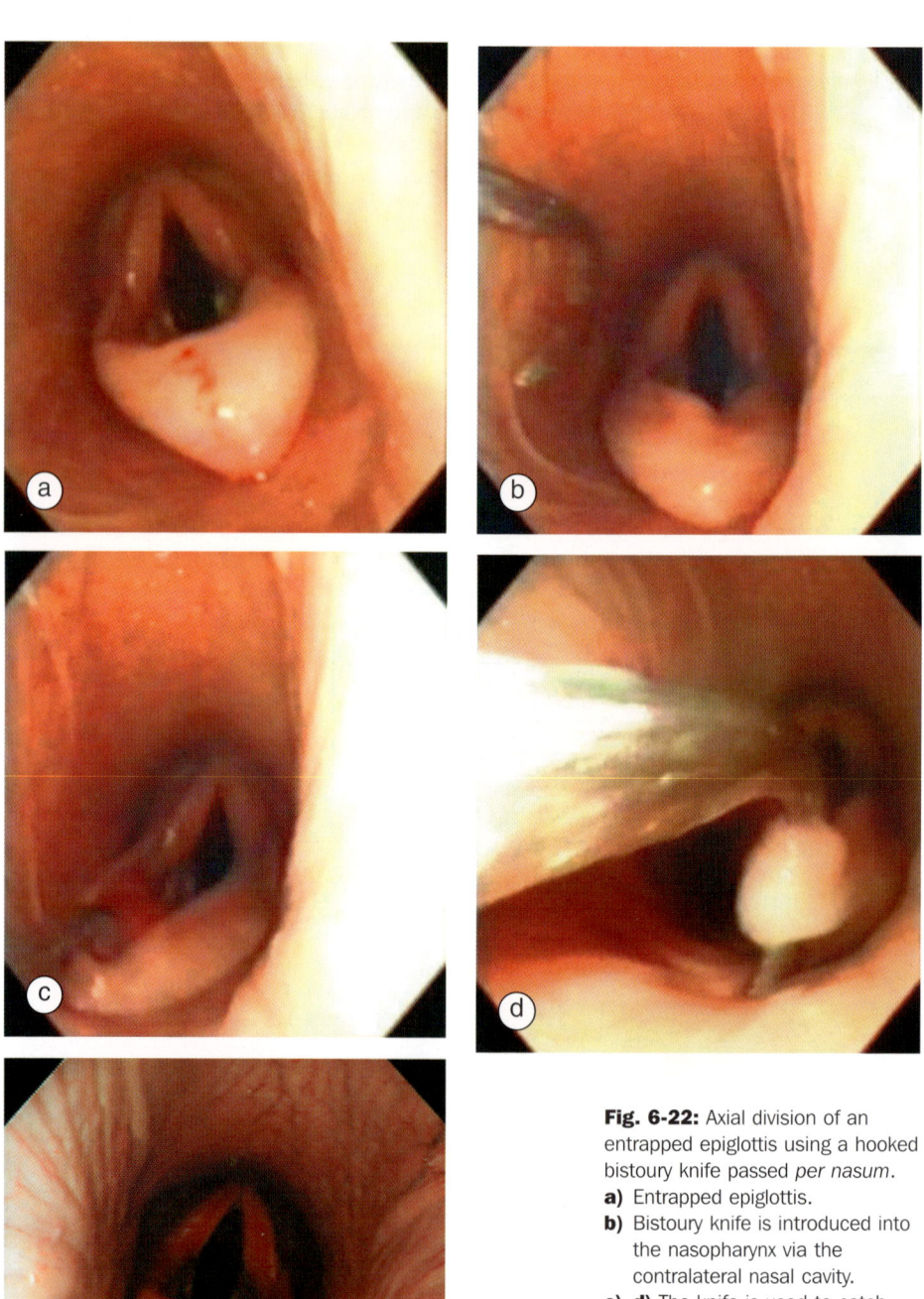

Fig. 6-22: Axial division of an entrapped epiglottis using a hooked bistoury knife passed *per nasum*.
a) Entrapped epiglottis.
b) Bistoury knife is introduced into the nasopharynx via the contralateral nasal cavity.
c), d) The knife is used to catch the entrapping fold and is then pulled rostrally, sectioning the entrapping mucosa whilst taking care not to damage the soft palate.
e) The mucosa has been divided, leaving the epiglottis free of entrapment.

Chapter 6: **Larynx**

Subepiglottic cysts

These lesions are most prevalent in young Thoroughbreds and Standardbreds, and are thought to be derived from the embryological remnants of the thryoglossal duct. Young foals with subepiglottic cysts may present with nasal reflux of milk, respiratory obstruction, and sometimes aspiration pneumonia. Less severely affected horses may not show clinical signs until they commence training, when they present with abnormal respiratory noise at exercise and exercise intolerance which may be attributable to secondary epiglottic retroflexion, epiglottic entrapment or persistent DDSP.

A subepiglottic cyst can be identified during endoscopic examination as a rounded mass positioned beneath the epiglottis, the tip of which is often abnormally dorsally angulated (Fig. 6-23). The cyst may be hidden from sight with the endoscope passed *per nasum*, because it has slipped below the soft palate, because the epiglottis is entrapped, or because persistent DDSP is present. In such cases inducing swallowing several times may transiently reveal the cyst. Alternatively, endoscopy performed *per os*, palpation of the subepiglottic area or a lateral radiograph of the laryngeal region may be of diagnostic value.

Treatment involves excision of the cyst via a laryngotomy, or using an electrocautery snare or transendoscopic laser surgery. Regardless of the method employed, all of the secretory lining of the cyst must be removed, or the cyst may re-form. Removal of an excessive amount of mucosa overlying the cyst must also be avoided because this may result in cicatrization of the subepiglottic tissues, causing intermittent or persistent DDSP.

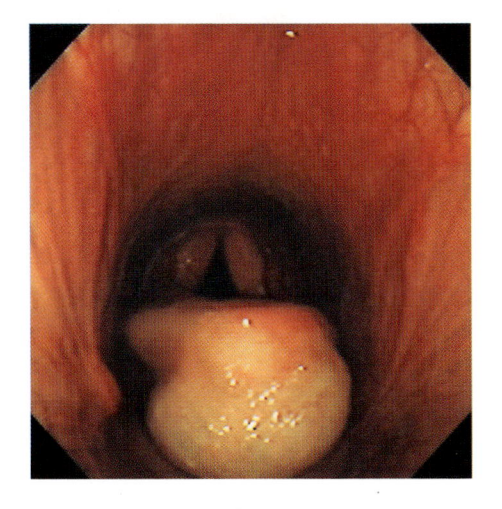

Fig. 6-23: Large subepiglottic cyst with associated epiglottal entrapment which is causing significant respiratory obstruction and dysphagia.

Epiglottitis (Fig. 6-24)

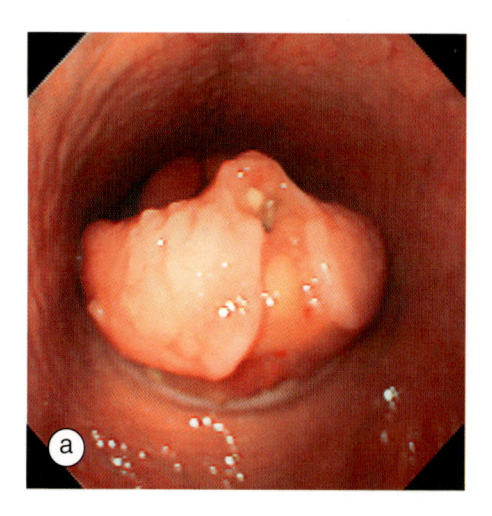

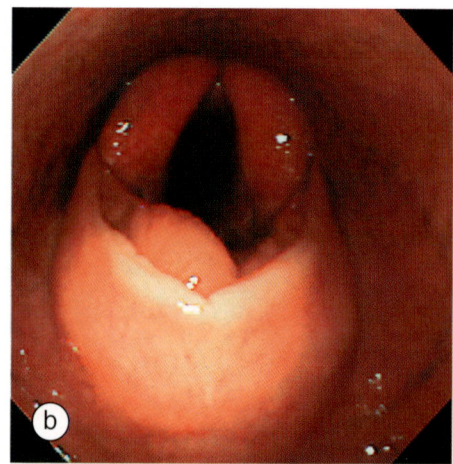

Epiglottitis occurs primarily in racehorses, and is thought to be caused by irritation and inflammatory changes due to repetitive trauma during exercise. The disorder is commonly associated with epiglottic entrapment. Affected horses make an abnormal respiratory noise at exercise, suffer from poor performance and cough excessively, particularly when eating. Most inflammatory changes involve the oral (ventral) epiglottic surface and the tip of the epiglottis. The epiglottic mucosa or the cartilage itself may be thickened and granulation tissue may be present. The normal ventral curvature of the epiglottis is often lost, and the epiglottic tip points dorsally. Treatment consists of rest and systemic and/or topical steroids and NSAIDs, but only 50% of affected racehorses are able to return to their previous level of performance. Horses may be left with a permanent epiglottic deformity after inflammation subsides.

Epiglottic hypoplasia/flaccidity

The term 'epiglottic hypoplasia' is often used confusingly to describe either an epiglottis that is short in length, thin or narrow, or an epiglottis which is normal in size, but appears to be flaccid.

Fig. 6-24: Epiglottitis.
a) The mucosa of the ventral epiglottis has been damaged and there is profound inflammation of the epiglottic cartilage.
b) Persistent DDSP is present in this horse, but the portion of the epiglottic cartilage which is visible above the ulcerated soft palate is thickened and edematous. Photograph courtesy of P. M. Dixon.

Chapter 6: Larynx

Lateral radiographs of a truly hypoplastic epiglottis confirm that the rostro-caudal length (from the apex of the epiglottis to the body of the thyroid cartilage) is shorter than the normal range (8.3–9.2 cm in a Thoroughbred).

The diagnosis of epiglottic flaccidity is subjective and is based on a 'flattened' appearance of the epiglottis during endoscopic examination (Fig. 6-25). It is often diagnosed in horses undergoing high-speed treadmill endoscopy, or during endoscopy of resting horses when the nostrils are occluded. However, a similar 'flattened' appearance of the epiglottis occurs after electrical stimulation of the hyoepiglotticus muscles. These muscles act to dilate the airway in exercising horses, and it is possible that dynamic epiglottal flaccidity observed during exercise or nasal occlusion may be a normal physiological reaction, and not a conformational abnormality of the epiglottis.

Epiglottic hypoplasia predisposes horses to develop epiglottal entrapment, but there are conflicting opinions as to whether epiglottic hypoplasia or flaccidity contribute towards intermittent DDSP. Many clinicians believe that there is a strong association between epiglottic hypoplasia/flaccidity and DDSP, but clinical and experimental evidence shows that the epiglottis is not required to maintain the palate in its normal position. Additionally, the length and appearance of the epiglottis in the majority of horses with intermittent DDSP is normal, and there is also no significant association between apparent epiglottic abnormalities and racing performance. Hence, it is questionable whether horses with epiglottic hypoplasia (without entrapment) actually require treatment. Epiglottic augmentation with submucosal injections of polytetrafluororoethylene (Teflon™) has been reported to be successful in increasing epiglottic size in horses with epiglottic hypoplasia and DDSP.

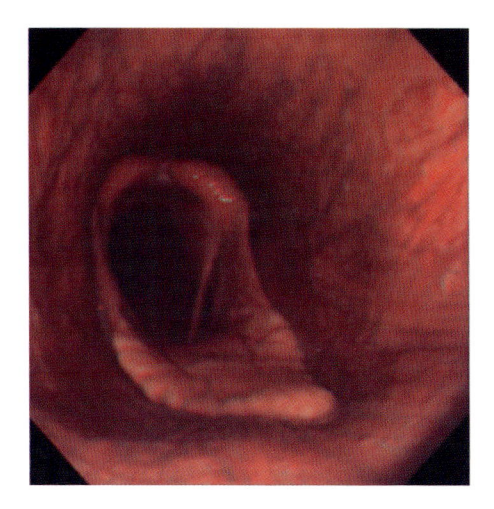

Fig. 6-25: Epiglottic flaccidity – the epiglottis in this horse is of normal length but appears flaccid, having lost its normal 'leaf-like' curvature. The significance of this finding is questionable, and this horse did not develop any other abnormalities during high-speed treadmill endoscopy. Photograph courtesy of P. Dixon.

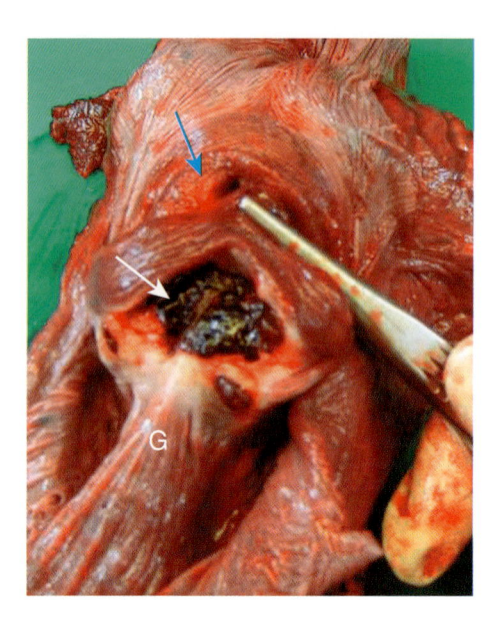

Fig. 6-26: Subepiglottic ulceration: cadaver larynx – the tip of the epiglottis is being retroverted with the forceps to reveal a large area of subepiglottic ulceration (white arrow). G = glossoepiglottic fold. This lesion would not be visible endoscopically unless the larynx was anesthetized and the epiglottis retroverted with a probe. The right arytenoid cartilage is just visible (blue arrow).

Subepiglottic ulceration

The etiology of subepiglottic ulceration is unknown. Possible causes are mucosal irritation caused by DDSP, infection of the respiratory tract, trauma to the tissue from foreign bodies during swallowing, or intermittent epiglottic entrapment. Indications for examining the subepiglottic area in the horse include abnormalities of the epiglottis, persistent DDSP, and abnormal respiratory noise during exercise or coughing when eating when no abnormalities are observed during routine endoscopy.

To examine this area, the horse must be sedated and the epiglottis anesthetized by topical application of local anesthetic solution. A curved probe with a blunt, forked end is then passed up the contralateral nostril to the endoscope, and used to retroflex the epiglottis in order to allow visualization of the subepiglottic tissues and the dorso-caudal border of the soft palate.

The most common lesion in this area is ulceration of the glossoepiglottic folds (Fig. 6-26), but excessive granulation tissue may also develop, and ulceration of the caudal border of the soft palate may also be observed. Affected horses are treated with rest and topical and/or systemic antibiotics combined with NSAIDs. Granulation tissue present may require resection using a transendoscopic laser.

Chapter 6: Larynx

FURTHER READING

Davenport-Goodall CL, Parente EJ 2003 Disorders of the larynx. Veterinary Clinics of North America Equine Practice 19:169–87

Dixon P 2006 Disorders of the larynx. In: Equine Respiratory Medicine and Surgery. Eds: McGorum, Robinson, Schumacher and Dixon. Saunders.

Dixon P, Robinson E, Wade JF (eds) 2004 Proceedings of a Workshop on Equine Recurrent Laryngeal Neuropathy. Havemeyer Foundation Monograph Series no. 11. R & W Publications, Newmarket

Hawkins JF, Tulleners EP 1994 Epiglottitis in horses: 20 cases (1988–1993). Journal of the American Veterinary Medical Association 205:1577–80

Kelly G, Lumsden JM, Dunkerly G et al. 2003 Idiopathic mucosal lesions of the arytenoid cartilages of 21 Thoroughbred yearlings: 1997–2001. Equine Veterinary Journal 35:276–81

Lane JG 2001 Fourth Branchial Arch Defects. Proceedings of the 2nd World Equine Airways Society Conference, Edinburgh, Scotland (CD-ROM)

Chapter preview

Normal anatomy 89

Tips for endoscopic examination 91

    Collection of tracheal secretions 93

    Collection of broncho-alveolar lavage (BAL) fluid 93

Abnormalities 94

    Pulmonary disease 94

    Exercise-induced pulmonary hemorrhage 94

    Tracheal collapse 97

    Tracheal neoplasia 99

    Tracheal obstruction following removal of tracheotomy tubes or tracheal trauma

    Dysphagia 101

    Tracheal trauma 101

    Thoracic venous congestion 102

    Foreign bodies 102

Further reading 102

7: Trachea and bronchi

Normal anatomy

The trachea extends from the larynx proximally to the carina distally. It is composed of 50–60 incomplete cartilaginous rings that are joined together by fibroelastic interannular ligaments. The incomplete dorsal aspect of the cartilage rings is bridged by the dorsal ligament and trachealis muscle. The trachea is lined with ciliated respiratory mucosa, within which are small blood vessels that are particularly prominent on the dorsal and lateral tracheal walls. The normal equine trachea is slightly flattened dorso-ventrally (Fig. 7-1), particularly the thoracic portion. The trachea of some normal horses may become more laterally flattened just proximal to the carina (Fig. 7-2).

Small, clinically insignificant, nodular cartilaginous protrusions may be present in the trachea of some horses, particularly in the ventral aspect of the cervical trachea (Fig. 7-3). Only a few flecks of mucus should be present in the trachea of normal horses. The tracheal 'sump' is the dependent horizontal portion of the cranial thoracic trachea (Fig. 7-4), and this is the area where excessive respiratory secretions tend to accumulate. It should be noted that if horses have traveled with their heads tied up immediately before tracheoscopy is performed, normal respiratory secretions may have accumulated due to reduced mucociliary clearance associated with the elevated head position.

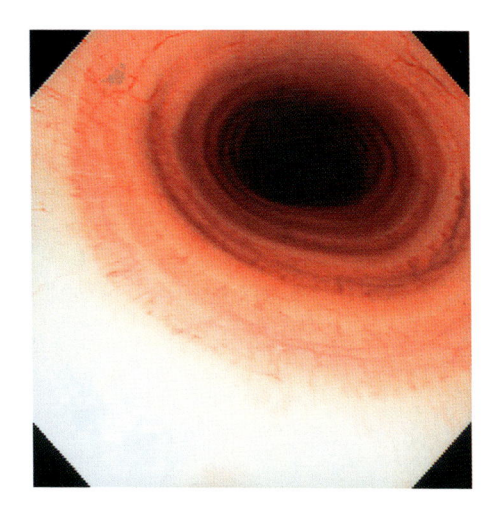

Fig. 7-1: Tracheal lumen in a normal horse. Note the slight dorso-ventral flattening which may become more apparent from the mid and distal cervical parts of the trachea.

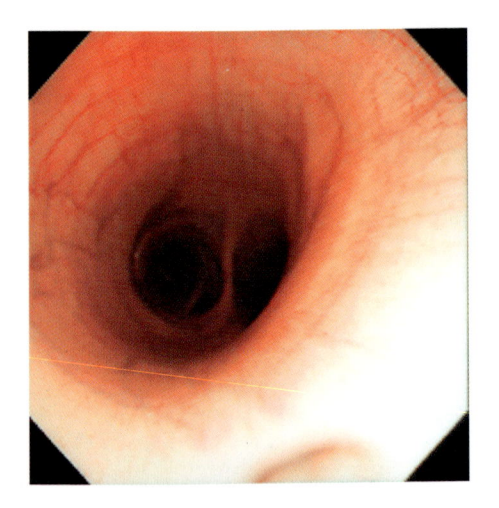

Fig. 7-2: The thoracic trachea may become laterally flattened in some normal horses just proximal to the carina.

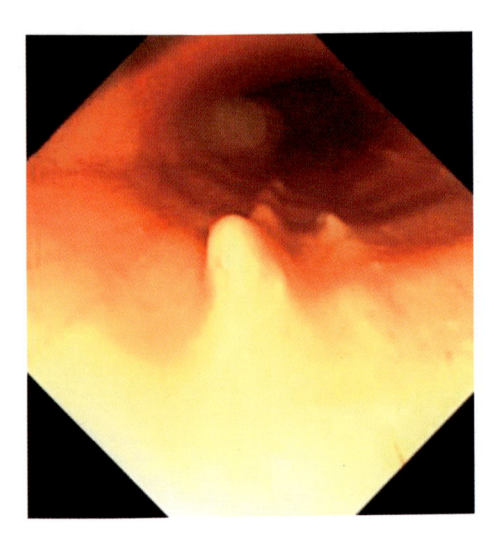

Fig. 7-3: Small cartilaginous protrusions in the upper cervical trachea are a normal variation in some horses. They are clinically insignificant.

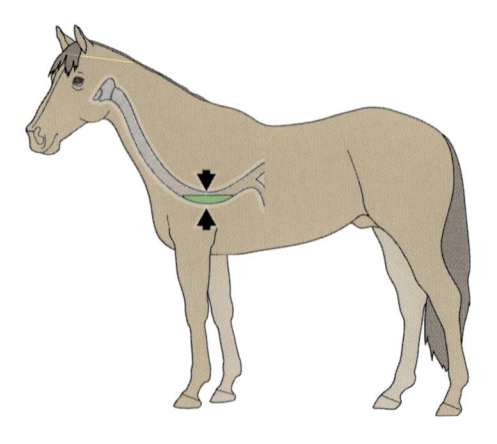

Fig. 7-4: Diagram showing the location of the tracheal 'sump' (arrows). This is the horizontal portion of the cranial thoracic trachea where respiratory secretions tend to accumulate and are readily sampled for tracheal aspirates/washes.

Chapter 7: **Trachea and bronchi**

The trachea divides into the left and right mainstem bronchi at the carina (Fig. 7-5). The right mainstem bronchus (Fig. 7-6) gives off the right cranial lobar bronchus laterally, then the right accessory lobar bronchus ventro-medially. The right caudal lobar first (ventrolaterally positioned) and second (dorso-laterally positioned) segmental bronchi branch off next, and the airway continues caudally as the right caudal lobar bronchus before dividing into several smaller segmental bronchi. The left mainstem bronchus (Fig. 7-7) shows a similar pattern of branching, except that there is no left accessory lobar bronchus.

Tips for endoscopic examination

A 100–110 cm endoscope is sufficiently long to allow examination of the proximal aspect of the trachea of adult horses, and to perform tracheal washes or collect aspirates. To examine the carina, the endoscope must be at least 140–160 cm long, and if bronchoscopy is to be performed, the diameter of the endoscope must additionally be narrow (10 mm or less). The proximal portion of the trachea is relatively insensitive unless inflamed, and can be examined endoscopically without the use of sedation or local anesthesia. However, sedatives (e.g. romifidine or detomidine with butorphanol) are required if broncho-alveolar lavage (BAL) is to be performed. The use of a topically applied local anesthetic solution does not make transendoscopic BAL significantly easier in most horses because coughing usually subsides within a few seconds after the endoscope is wedged in position. If extensive bronchoscopy is to be performed, topical application of local anesthetic solution to the bronchial mucosa will reduce the cough reflex so that the endoscope can be moved into different areas of the bronchial tree.

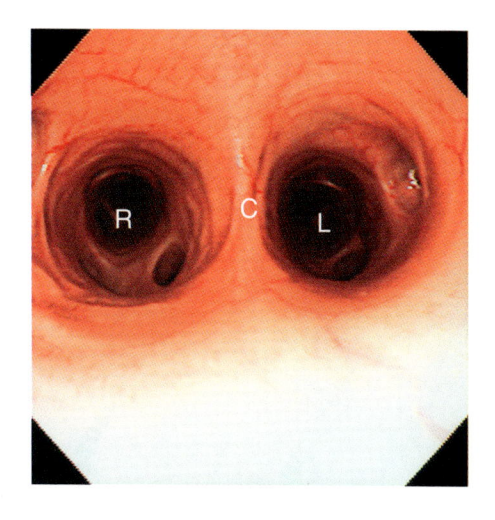

Fig. 7-5: View of the carina in a normal horse. The left (L) and right (R) mainstem bronchi can be seen, with smaller bronchial branches in the distance. Note the 'sharp' appearance of the carina (C).

Handbook of Equine Respiratory Endoscopy

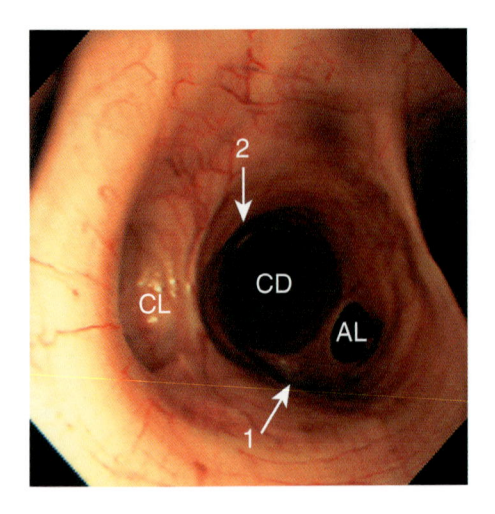

Fig. 7-6: Right mainstem bronchus showing right cranial lobar bronchus (CL), right accessory lobar bronchus (AL), right first (1) and second (2) segmental bronchi and right caudal lobar bronchus (CD).

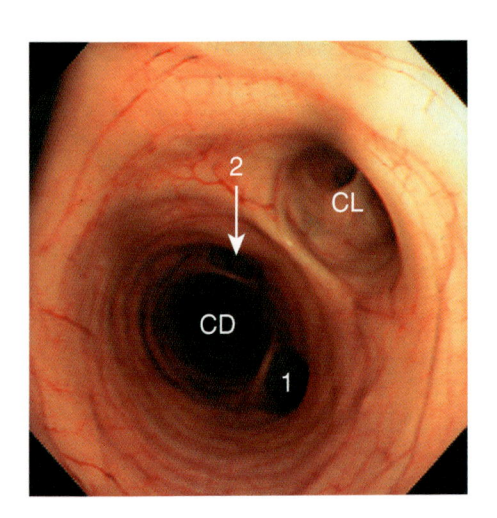

Fig. 7-7: Left mainstem bronchus showing left cranial lobar bronchus (CL), left first (1) and second (2) segmental bronchi and left caudal lobar bronchus (CD).

Table 7-1: Comparison of tracheal wash with broncho-alveolar lavage

	Tracheal wash	Broncho-alveolar lavage
Length of endoscope required	100–110 cm	160 cm (or BAL catheter)
Sedation required	No	Yes
Collected sample represents cytology of all lower airways?	Yes	No – only one part of the lung is sampled
Quality of cell morphology at cytological examination	Variable	Excellent
Post-procedure exercise regime	As normal	No fast work for 48 hours

Chapter 7: **Trachea and bronchi**

The relative merits and disadvantages of performing tracheal washes and broncho-alveolar lavage (BAL) are summarized in Table 7-1. The author routinely performs both when investigating cases of lower respiratory disease, unless the horse is due to race under rules, because the use of sedative drugs precludes racing until the relevant drug withdrawal times have passed.

Collection of tracheal secretions

If a large volume of tracheal secretions are present in the 'sump' of the trachea, it is usually possible to aspirate a sample using a transendoscopic aspiration/delivery catheter. A guarded catheter (Fig. 1-07) should be used if the sample is to be sent for bacteriological culture, as this prevents bacteria from the upper respiratory tract contaminating the sample. If only a small amount of respiratory secretions are present, or if the secretions are too thick to be easily aspirated, a tracheal wash can be performed. This involves the instillation of approximately 10 ml of warmed sterile physiological saline solution into the proximal part of the trachea, before passing the endoscope down to the sump and aspirating the pooled fluid (Fig. 7-8).

Collection of broncho-alveolar lavage (BAL) fluid

BAL fluid can be collected using a proprietary BAL catheter (e.g. Fogarty catheter or Bivona cuffed BAL catheter) with an inflatable cuff at the distal end, or using a long endoscope. Benefits of the transendoscopic technique include a higher incidence of success, the ability to select a particular bronchus for BAL and a low incidence of iatrogenic airway hemorrhage, resulting in less blood contamination of the sample. The transendoscopic technique involves guiding the tip of the endoscope into the right accessory lobar bronchus; the accessory lobar bronchus is selected because the tip of a 160 cm endoscope can consistently reach this bronchus in most sizes of horses (Fig. 7-6). The horse often coughs a few times as the endoscope is introduced past the carina because the carina is richly innervated with cough receptors, but in most cases the cough is transient. The tip of the scope is then 'wedged' in

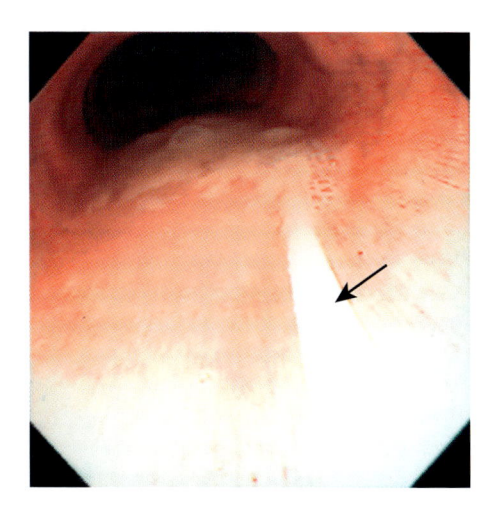

Fig. 7-8: Horse undergoing a tracheal wash – 10 ml of saline has been instilled into the proximal trachea, which has now accumulated in the tracheal sump with the respiratory secretions, and is being aspirated using a simple transendoscopic catheter (arrow).

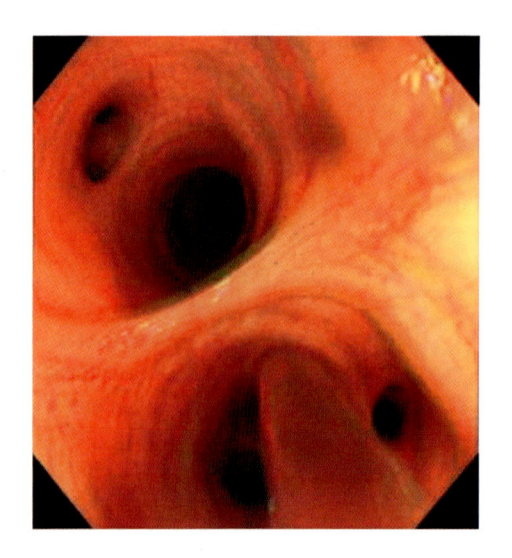

Fig. 7-9: Instillation of warmed saline into the branches of right accessory lobar bronchus during broncho-alveolar lavage. The tip of the endoscope is 'wedged' into the bronchus, forming an airtight seal.

the right accessory lobar bronchus, to form an airtight seal. Once the tip is wedged, 200 ml of warmed sterile physiological saline is instilled into the right accessory lobe via the biopsy channel of the endoscope (Fig. 7-9). This fluid is then immediately aspirated using large (50 ml) syringes. Recovery of less than 50% of the volume of fluid instilled is normal. Complete failure to recover fluid is most commonly caused by movement of the endoscope into another bronchus at some point during the procedure due to the horse coughing. Complications of transendoscopic BAL are rare and transient but include mild airway hyperemia, mild airway hemorrhage, pyrexia and pulmonary neutrophilia.

Abnormalities

Pulmonary disease

Horses with pulmonary disease such as heaves, inflammatory airway disease, pulmonary infection or neoplasia usually accumulate excessive mucopurulent or purulent respiratory secretions in the tracheal sump (Fig. 7-10), due to both excessive production of mucus and reduced mucociliary transport. These secretions may transiently cover the walls of the trachea instead of remaining in a pool if a horse has just coughed. The carina may have a 'blunted' appearance if the mucosal lining of the respiratory tract is inflamed (Fig. 7-11).

Exercise-induced pulmonary hemorrhage (Fig. 7-12a, b)

Exercise-induced pulmonary hemorrhage (EIPH) may occur in up to 95% of Thoroughbred racehorses in training (as diagnosed by tracheal wash cytology). The precise etiology of EIPH is currently unknown, but hypotheses include:

- Stress failure of pulmonary capillaries resulting from increased intrapulmonary pressures and simultaneously increased pulmonary arterial blood pressure.

- Trauma to the dorso-caudal lungs induced by locomotory impact during fast work.

Chapter 7: **Trachea and bronchi**

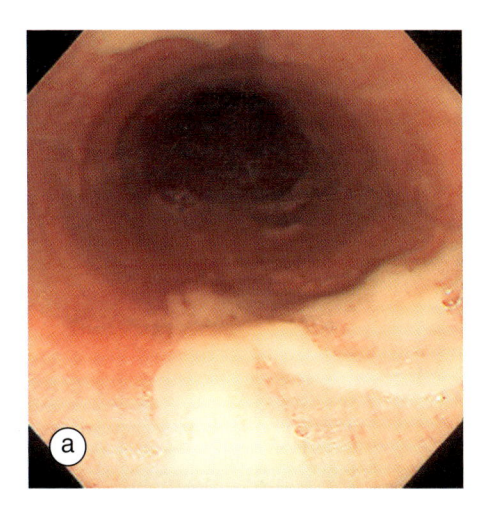

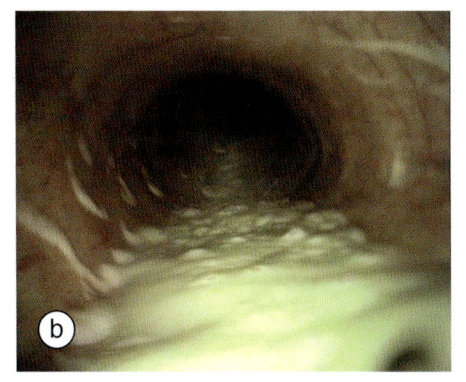

Fig. 7-10: Horses with heaves.
a) Moderate and
b) large pool of mucopurulent respiratory secretions accumulated in the 'sump' of the trachea.

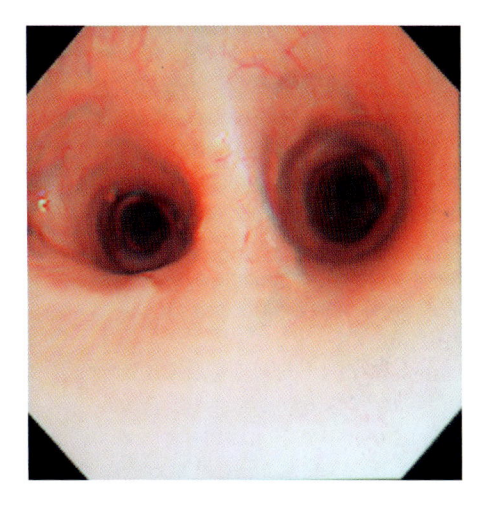

Fig. 7-11: Horse with lower airway disease and a 'blunted' appearance to the carina due to mucosal inflammation.

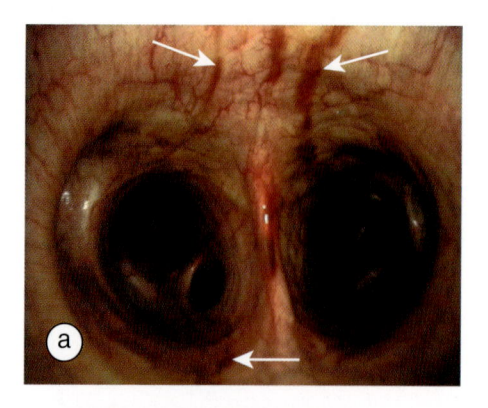

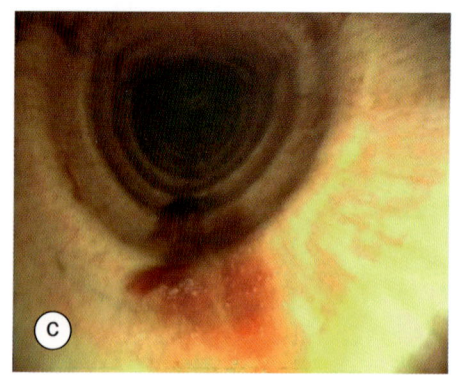

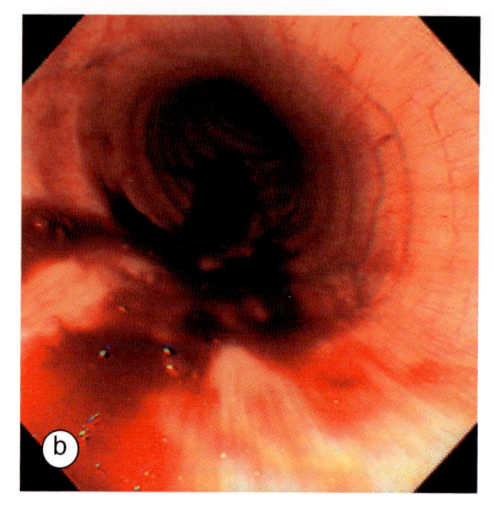

Fig. 7-12: Exercise-induced pulmonary hemorrhage.
a) Grade 1: small amount of blood (arrows) emanating from the mainstem bronchi, photograph courtesy of J. Keen.
b) Grade 3: continuous stream of blood which is less than half the tracheal width.
c) Brown-tinged tracheal secretions in a horse that had severe EIPH several days previously. Photograph courtesy of J. Keen.

The role of chronic inflammation of the lower airways in the etiopathogenesis of EIPH is controversial, because it is not clear whether the lower airway inflammation seen commonly in horses with EIPH is a cause or result of the bleeding. Many horses with EIPH show no clinical signs, with only 1 out of 10 affected horses exhibiting epistaxis. Other affected horses may perform poorly or cough. If only a small volume of pulmonary hemorrhage is present, epistaxis may be unilateral or may occur only when the horse lowers its head. EIPH can be diagnosed with reasonable certainty in horses which exhibit epistaxis after fast exercise, but in the majority of cases the disease is diagnosed during endoscopic examination. Blood is most likely to be visualized in the trachea 60–90 minutes after fast work, and its appearance may vary from a large stream to thin streaks on the walls of the trachea, emanating from the primary bronchi. A semi-quantitative grading system for EIPH is shown in Table 7-2. Brown, discolored blood may be present in the trachea for weeks after the episode, if hemorrhage has been severe (Fig 7-12c).

Tracheal aspirates or BAL fluid samples obtained from affected horses may be pink or brown-tinged. In the acute stage, erythrocytes can be seen on cytological examination of these samples, either free or within phagocytosing macrophages. Hemosiderophages will be present in respiratory secretions for weeks to months after a single episode of EIPH.

Chapter 7: Trachea and bronchi

Table 7-2: Grading system for exercise induced pulmonary hemorrhage (EIPH)

Grade	Endoscopic examination of trachea
1	Flecks of blood only
2	> Flecks < continuous stream
3	Bloodstream < half tracheal width
4	Bloodstream > half tracheal width
5	Airways filled with blood

Treatments for horses which have experienced a severe episode of EIPH include rest and administration of an NSAID to allow resolution of lung inflammation, use of a graded incremental training regime, intravenous administration of frusemide prior to fast work, use of nasal strips, treatment of chronic lower airway inflammation and investigation and treatment of concurrent upper airway disorders.

Tracheal collapse

Tracheal collapse occurs primarily in small pony breeds (e.g. Shetland ponies) and donkeys and is caused by flaccidity of the dorsal ligaments (Fig. 7-13), deformity of the tracheal cartilages (Fig. 7-14a) or separation of the tracheal mucosa from the dorsal ligament of the tracheal rings. The distal cervical or thoracic trachea is most commonly involved, but occasionally the mainstem bronchi are affected. Clinical signs may go unnoticed in some affected ponies, due to their sedentary lifestyle, but in most cases stridor and dyspnea are observed at rest or during exercise and may worsen as the pony ages.

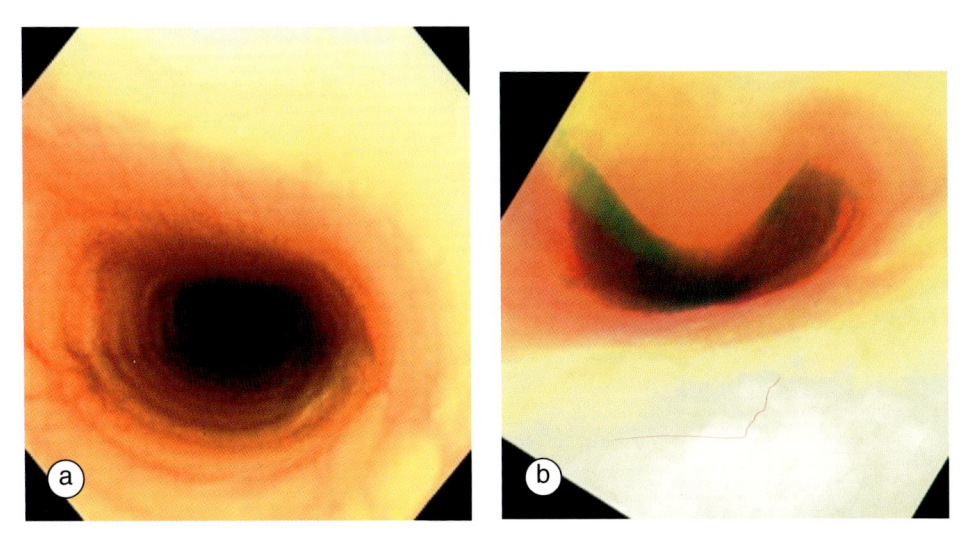

Fig. 7-13: Tracheal collapse. Distal cervical trachea of a 7-year-old Shetland pony during **a)** expiration and **b)** inspiration showing inspiratory collapse of the dorsal trachea due to flaccidity of the dorsal ligaments.

Tracheal collapse can be confirmed using radiography or endoscopy. The tracheal lumen of the cervical trachea of normal horses reduces mildly in diameter during inspiration, due to the negative pressures exerted at this stage in the respiratory cycle, but this effect is usually negligible. Lateral radiographs of affected ponies taken during expiration often appear normal, but those taken during inspiration show marked narrowing of the air column within the trachea at the site of obstruction (Fig. 7-14b). Palpation of the trachea may reveal abnormally shaped cartilages in some ponies. Endoscopic examination of the trachea of affected ponies reveals collapse of the cervical trachea during inspiration, which may become worse when the nostrils are temporarily occluded.

Tracheal collapse may also occur after traumatic damage to cartilage rings, or if several tracheal rings were completely transected during placement of a tracheotomy tube. The intrathoracic portion of the trachea may also undergo transient collapse in horses affected with severe pulmonary diseases as a result of raised intrathoracic pressures.

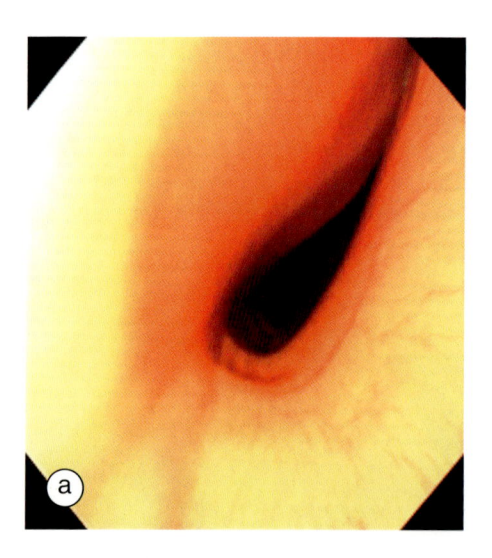

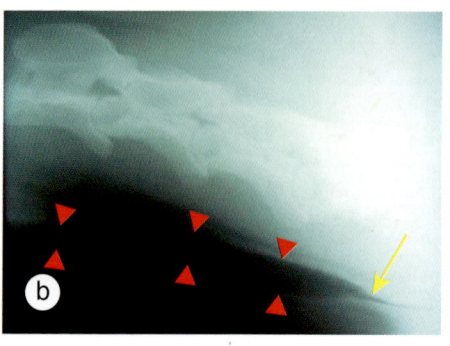

Fig. 7-14: Tracheal collapse secondary to deformity of tracheal cartilages in a Shetland pony.
a) Endoscopy of the trachea shows the abnormal shape of the lumen.
b) Radiograph taken during inspiration. The normal wide lumen of the proximal cervical trachea (red arrowheads) narrows markedly in the caudal cervical region (yellow arrow).

Chapter 7: **Trachea and bronchi**

Tracheal neoplasia

Primary neoplastic conditions of the trachea and bronchi are rare but include tracheal 'polyps' (Fig. 7-15), lymphoma, squamous cell carcinoma, chondroma (Fig. 7-16) and myxoma. Treatment may not be feasible if a large portion of the trachea is involved, but solitary benign growths can sometimes be excised through a tracheotomy incision, or transendoscopically using a snare or a laser.

Neoplastic cervical or intrathoracic masses that are located near to the trachea may impinge on the trachea and cause extra luminal tracheal obstruction (Fig. 7-17).

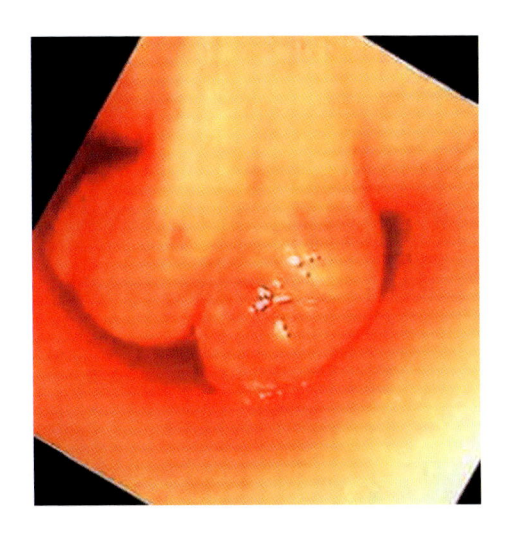

Fig. 7-15: Large tracheal polyp. This horse presented with progressively worsening stridor and dyspnea which became more severe at exercise or when the horse was stressed.

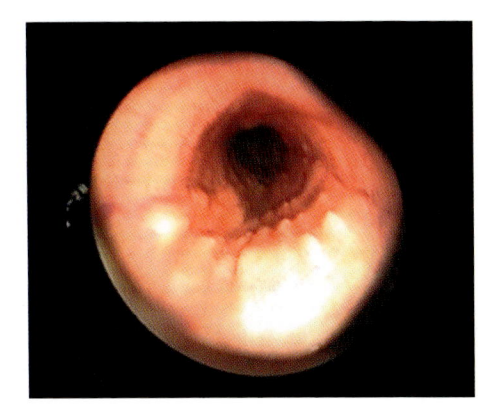

Fig. 7-16: Tracheal chondroma. This horse presented with clinical signs of lower airway disease and on endoscopy, this proliferative lesion could be seen along the entire length of the trachea and extending into the primary bronchi. Biopsy and histopathology of this lesion revealed it to be a tracheal chondroma. Photograph courtesy of T. Leaman.

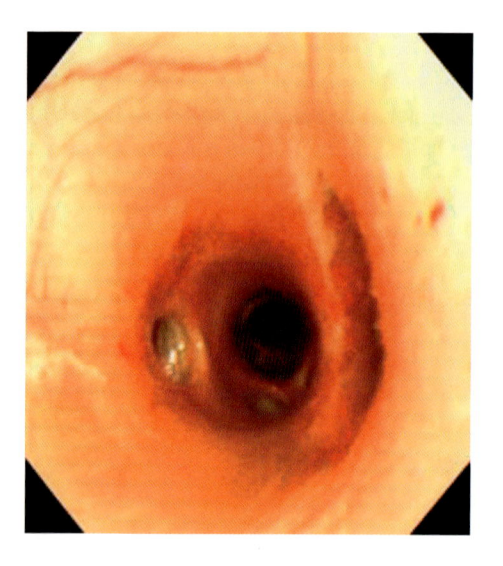

Fig. 7-17: Extraluminal tracheal obstruction. Distal trachea and carina of a 7-year-old pony with an intrathoracic lymphosarcoma which is impinging on the left side of the distal trachea, almost completely obstructing the left mainstem bronchus. The carina is inflamed and has a blunt appearance. Photograph courtesy of J. Keen.

Tracheal obstruction following removal of tracheotomy tubes or tracheal trauma

Damaged tracheal mucosa usually heals without complications, but occasionally, excessive intraluminal granulation tissue may develop (e.g. at a tracheotomy site [Fig. 7-18], or after traumatic injury to the trachea), and may cause significant obstruction to airflow. The horse may be left with a tracheal stricture when the granulation tissue remodels and contracts. Treatment is aimed at removal of excessive granulation tissue, which is most commonly performed transendoscopically using a laser.

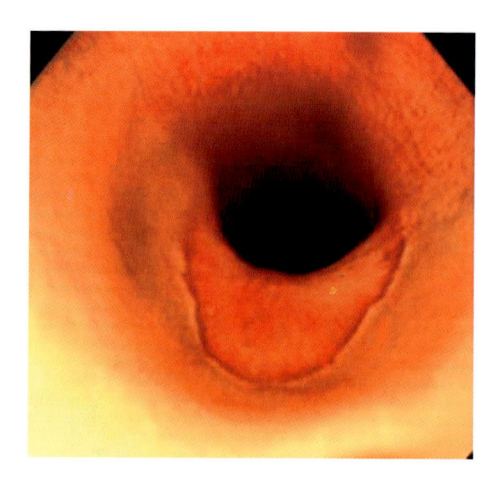

Fig. 7-18: Tracheal stenosis. Trachea 5 weeks after removal of a tracheotomy tube. The lumen is narrowed at the tracheotomy site, caused by excessive intraluminal granulation tissue.

Chapter 7: **Trachea and bronchi**

Dysphagia

Dysphagic horses, such as those with esophageal obstruction or pharyngeal paralysis, or those recovering from laryngeal surgery, may accumulate saliva or food material in the trachea and bronchi (Fig. 7-19). Saliva can be distinguished from respiratory secretions by its particularly white color and foamy, tenacious appearance.

Tracheal trauma

Kick wounds to the ventral aspect of the neck may result in tracheal perforation or deformation (Fig. 7-20). Horses with perforation of the tracheal mucosa experience leakage of air into the tissues of the neck, and subcutaneous emphysema quickly develops. Emphysema may spread to the head, causing respiratory obstruction in severe cases, or may cause pneumomediastinum, which can lead to a life-threatening pneumothorax if large amounts of air migrate through the mediastinum and into the pleural cavity.

If the tracheal wound is located in the upper cervical trachea, placing a tracheotomy tube distal to the wound will prevent emphysema from worsening by bypassing the injured area. If this is not possible, conservative treatment consisting of box rest and administration of tetanus antitoxin, NSAIDs and antibiotics should be instigated.

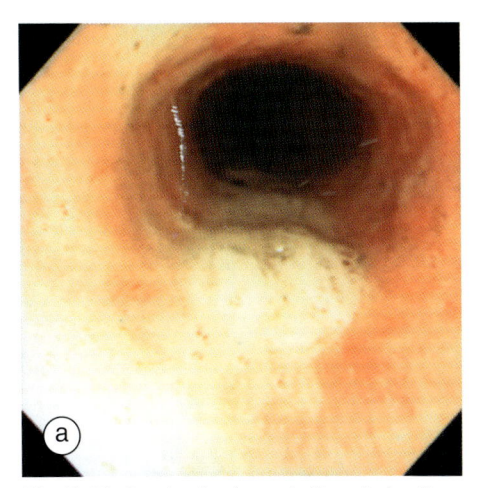

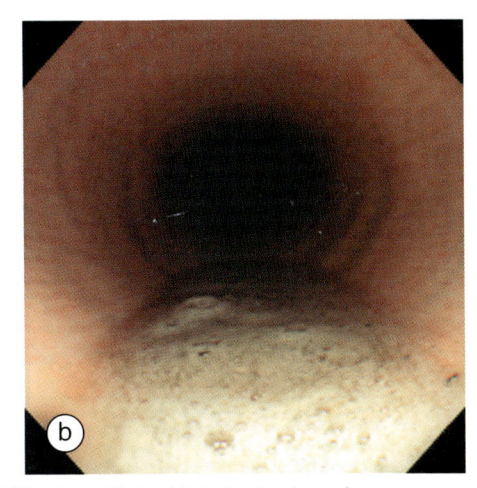

Fig. 7-19: Dysphagia. An aspiration of **a)** saliva and **b)** saliva with food into the trachea after prosthetic laryngoplasty (tie-back) operations. Note the white, foamy, tenacious appearance of the saliva.

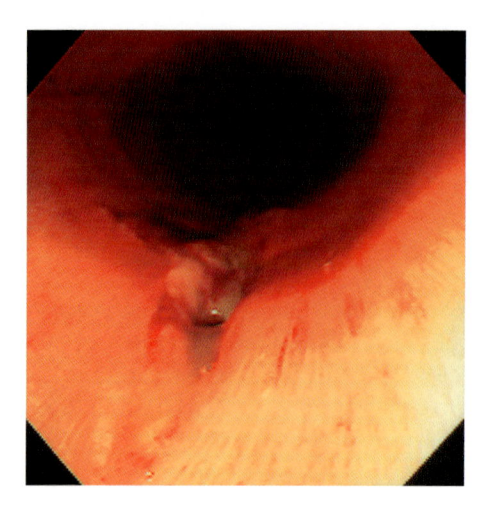

Fig. 7-20: Perforating injury of the trachea. This horse sustained a traumatic injury to its ventral neck, resulting in a small perforation of the tracheal mucosa. Transient emphysema of the neck developed, but the mucosal defect healed without other complications.

Thoracic venous congestion

Horses in congestive heart failure or horses experiencing obstruction to the thoracic vessels (e.g. due to space-occupying masses in the anterior mediastinum) may have particularly prominent tracheal veins visible on the lateral aspects of the trachea. Severely affected horses may have frothy serous fluid in the trachea, emanating from the bronchial tree.

Foreign bodies

Inhaled foreign bodies rarely reach the lower airways of horses, but if they do, clinical signs may include sudden onset of paroxysmal coughing and mucopurulent nasal discharge. Foreign bodies may be difficult to visualize endoscopically, due to inflammation of traumatized and infected mucosa and copious amounts of respiratory secretions. Removal can usually be performed using transendoscopic biopsy forceps or via a tracheotomy incision.

FURTHER READING

Birks EK, Durando MM, McBride S 2003 Exercise-induced pulmonary hemorrhage. Veterinary Clinics of North America Equine Practice 19:87–100

Dixon PM, Railton DI, McGorum BC 1995 Equine pulmonary disease: a case control study of 300 referred cases. Part 3: Ancillary diagnostic findings. Equine Veterinary Journal 27:428–35

Freeman DE 1989 Wounds of the esophagus and trachea. Veterinary Clinics of North America Equine Practice 5:683–93

Hoffman AM, Viel L 1997 Techniques for sampling the respiratory tract of horses. Veterinary Clinics of North America Equine Practice 13:463–75

Chapter preview

Introduction 105

Normal anatomy 106

Abnormalities 107
  Intermittent dorsal displacement of the soft palate (DDSP) and palatal instability
  Recurrent laryngeal neuropathy (RLN) 108
  Intermittent epiglottic entrapment 111
  Axial deviation of the aryepiglottic folds (ADAF) 112
  Nasopharyngeal collapse 113
  Fourth branchial arch defects (4-BAD, cricopharyngeal-laryngeal dysplasia) 115
  Epiglottic retroversion and axial collapse of the lateral margins of the epiglottis
  Bilateral arytenoid cartilage and vocal fold collapse 116
  Collapse of the apex of the corniculate process of the left arytenoid cartilage 1
  Multiple abnormalities 117

Further reading 117

8: High-speed treadmill endoscopy

Introduction

High-speed treadmill endoscopy (HSTE) is an indispensable tool for assessing the upper respiratory tract of equine athletes. The use of HSTE has provided clinicians with a means for accurately identifying dynamic causes of upper airway obstruction that are not observed in horses at rest, such as intermittent dorsal displacement of the soft palate (DDSP), vocal fold or arytenoid cartilage collapse, nasopharyngeal collapse, axial deviation of the aryepiglottic folds, intermittent epiglottal entrapment, and epiglottic retroversion.
At exercise, the volume of air moving through the upper respiratory tract increases dramatically (from 4 L/second in a resting horse to approximately 75 L/second in a galloping horse). To meet the horse's increased oxygen requirement and move such large volumes of air into the lungs, large negative pressures must be generated within the respiratory tract during inspiration. These negative pressures tend to collapse the non-rigid parts of the upper airway such as the nasopharynx and larynx, and active muscular effort is required to resist collapse and maintain an adequate, functional airway. Failure of the non-rigid parts of the upper respiratory tract to resist negative inspiratory pressures results in 'dynamic' obstruction during exercise.

High-speed treadmill endoscopic examinations require experienced personnel and expensive equipment, and are therefore only available at specialist centers. The endoscope can be attached to the horse's halter using Velcro straps or a Penrose drain. High-quality videoendoscopic equipment with either digital or video recording is essential for performing HSTE, because the rapid movements of the nasopharynx and larynx are often seen more clearly during slow-motion playback. To examine racehorses, the treadmill must be capable of attaining speeds of up to 14 m/s and inclining 3–10° uphill (Fig. 8-1). The use of an incline allows the animal to perform increased work effort at submaximal speeds. A full clinical examination including examination for lameness should be performed before any horse is exercised on a treadmill, to rule out conditions that may render the horse

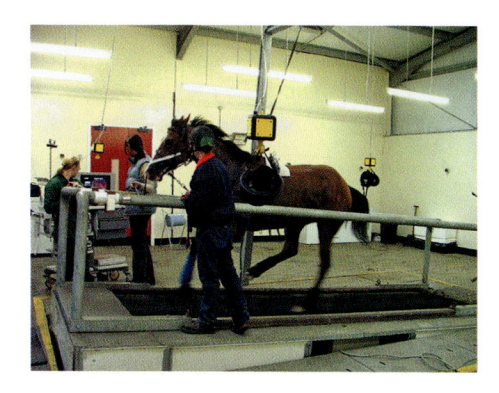

Fig. 8-1: Racehorse undergoing HSTE. Note the uphill incline of the treadmill, used to increase the workload at submaximal speeds.

unsuitable for fast exercise. The horse should always be endoscopically examined while at rest first, because this may reveal obvious structural or functional abnormalities that negate the need for a HSTE examination. Horses usually require 1–3 treadmill training sessions before it is safe to perform HSTE.

The high-speed treadmill does not completely reproduce racing conditions and even when horses are taken to the point of fatigue on a treadmill, the level of exertion may not replicate that of a race. Factors such as the weight of the jockey, varying underfoot conditions, and the excitement or stress of race day cannot be exactly reproduced, and this may explain why an endoscopic diagnosis may not be achieved during HSTE of some horses with a history of abnormal respiratory noise and poor performance during racing. Additional techniques that can be performed on horses undergoing HSTE include exercise electrocardiograms, recording of respiratory noises, measurement of intrapharyngeal and intratracheal pressures, analysis of respiratory gases, arterial and venous blood samples, and high-speed gait analysis.

Normal anatomy

During exercise, both arytenoid cartilages should attain and maintain full abduction with no deviation from this position, apart from during swallowing, until ventilation returns to resting levels (Fig. 8-2). The roof of the nasopharynx may displace ventrally at the end of expiration and this finding should be considered to be within normal limits if it does not obstruct more than one-third of the rima glottidis. The horse remains able to swallow during strenuous exercise, during which full adduction of both arytenoids will transiently occur, followed by a rapid return to the fully abducted position. During swallowing, the action of the circular muscles of the pharyngeal walls causes the pharynx to constrict transiently. Normal horses may swallow several times, particularly at the beginning of exercise, but repeated swallowing throughout an exercise test may indicate the presence of an irritating stimulus in the upper respiratory tract.

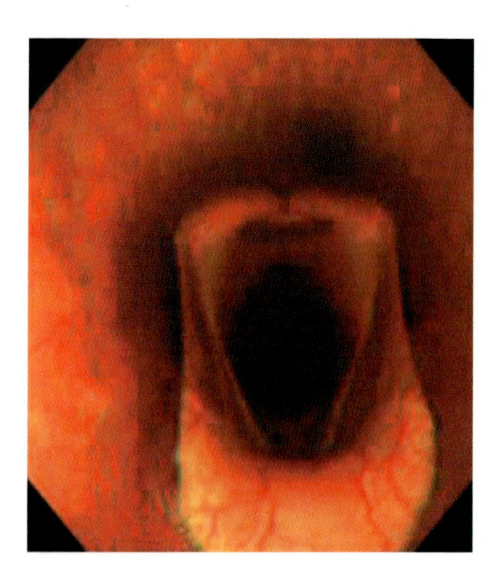

Fig. 8-2: Normal endoscopic appearance of the equine larynx during exercise (grade A laryngeal function during exercise). Note both arytenoid cartilages are fully and symmetrically abducted, the vocal folds and aryepiglottic folds are not collapsing axially and the epiglottis is dorsal to the soft palate.

Chapter 8: **High-speed treadmill endoscopy**

Abnormalities

Intermittent dorsal displacement of the soft palate (DDSP) and palatal instability

Intermittent DDSP is the most commonly diagnosed cause of upper airway obstruction in horses undergoing HSTE examination for investigation of poor performance. Horses that

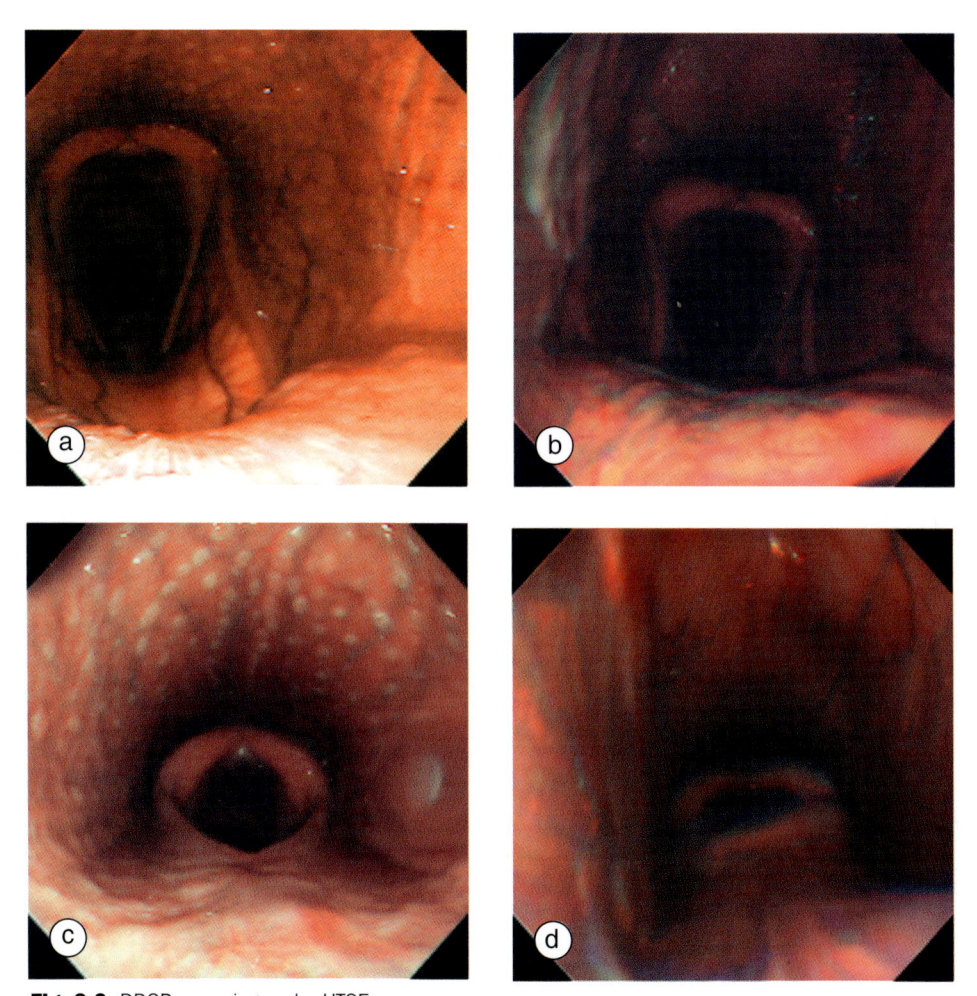

Fig. 8-3: DDSP occurring under HTSE.
- **a)** The epiglottis appears to 'flatten' against the dorsal aspect of the soft palate. Note the full and symmetrical abduction of both arytenoid cartilages.
- **b)** Palatal instability – the palate undergoes wave-like 'billowing'. Mild axial deviation of the right aryepiglottic fold is also evident in this photograph.
- **c)** DDSP – the palate has displaced dorsal to the epiglottis and is causing obstruction of the rima glottis.
- **d)** The obstruction becomes worse during expiration as the caudal border of the palate is lifted further dorsally.

dorsally displace their soft palates during nasal occlusion at rest do not necessarily experience DDSP while exercising, and conversely, some horses that do not displace their soft palates during nasal occlusion at rest do develop DDSP during exercise. Palatal instability (Fig. 8-3b), seen as 'billowing' of the soft palate without displacement of its caudal border, causes turbulent airflow within the nasopharynx and commonly precedes DDSP. This wave-like billowing begins at the junction of the hard and soft palates, and progresses caudally. As the soft palate 'billows' dorsally, it may lift the epiglottis and in turn cause the aryepiglottic folds to deviate axially to some degree before the soft palate displaces dorsally (Fig. 8-3b).

The dorsally displaced soft palate causes a marked obstruction of the rima glottidis (Fig. 8-3d) and many affected horses make a loud expiratory 'gurgle' and are usually unable to continue exercising at high speed. Clinically normal horses may occasionally transiently displace their soft palates at exercise, but a normal horse typically swallows and very quickly replaces the palate to a subepiglottic position.

The proposed etiology of DDSP and treatment of affected horses are discussed in Chapter 4.

Recurrent laryngeal neuropathy (RLN)

Recurrent laryngeal neuropathy is the second most commonly diagnosed cause of upper airway obstruction in horses undergoing HSTE examination for investigation of poor performance. Endoscopic grading of laryngeal function with the horse at rest is described in Chapter 6. Endoscopic grading of laryngeal function during exercise can be categorized as grade A (Fig. 8-2), B (Figs 8-4, 8-5) or C (Fig. 8-6), and definitions of these grades are shown in Table 8-1.

The endoscopic grade of laryngeal function at rest (1–4) usually indicates what is likely to occur at exercise, with the majority of resting grade 1 and 2 horses (i.e. those that are able to attain and maintain full bilateral arytenoid abduction) being classified as grade A at exercise, and all those with grade 4 laryngeal function at rest being classified as grade C at exercise. Occasionally, horses with grade 1 or 2 laryngeal function at rest may experience some degree of collapse of the arytenoid cartilage or vocal fold during HSTE and therefore dynamic RLN cannot be completely ruled out on the basis of resting endoscopic findings alone. Clinicians who do not have facilities for treadmill testing should therefore not immediately discount RLN as a potential cause of abnormal respiratory noise during exercise if a horse has grade 1 or 2 laryngeal function at rest.

High-speed treadmill endoscopic examination of horses with grade 3 laryngeal function at rest allows differentiation between horses that do and do not experience dynamic laryngeal collapse. If laryngeal collapse does occur, HSTE may also guide the surgeon as to which surgical procedure is the most suitable. Published reports from different centres vary markedly in the proportions of horses with grade 3 laryngeal function at rest which are classified as grade A (4–48%), grade B (15–82%) or grade C (15–77%) during maximal exercise. Horses with significant dynamic arytenoid collapse require a laryngoplasty and ventriculocordectomy or a neuromuscular pedicle graft if they are to perform athletically. The vocal fold and laryngeal ventricle of some horses with grade A or B laryngeal function at

Chapter 8: High-speed treadmill endoscopy

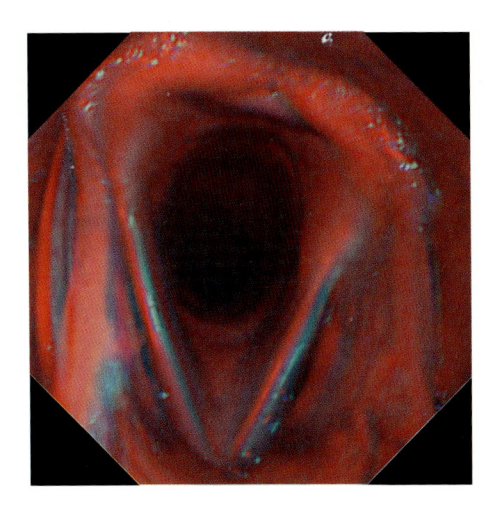

Fig. 8-4: Grade B laryngeal function in the exercising horse – the left arytenoid is not fully abducted. There is no vocal fold collapse. There is mild axial deviation of the right ary-epiglottic fold.

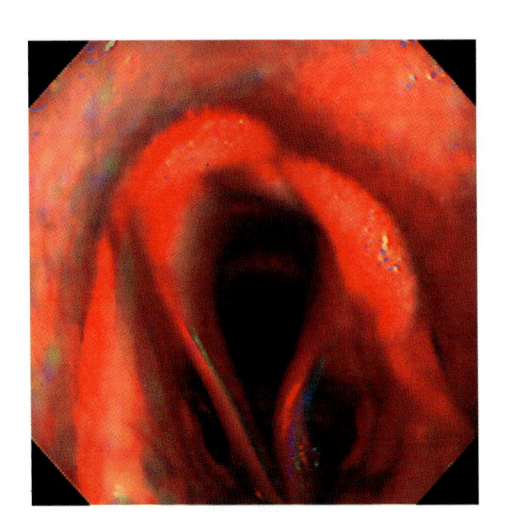

Fig. 8-5: Grade B laryngeal function in an exercising horse – the left arytenoid is only partially abducted and there is also marked axial collapse of the left vocal fold.

Table 8-1: Grading system for assessment of laryngeal function in the horse during exercise

Laryngeal grade	Definition
A	Full abduction of the arytenoid cartilages during inspiration
B	Partial abduction of the affected arytenoid cartilage (between full abduction and the resting position)
C	Abduction less than resting position including collapse of the affected arytenoid cartilage into the contralateral half of the rima glottidis during inspiration

Source: Proceedings of the Havemeyer Foundation Workshop on Equine Recurrent Laryngeal Neuropathy, p 97

Handbook of Equine Respiratory Endoscopy

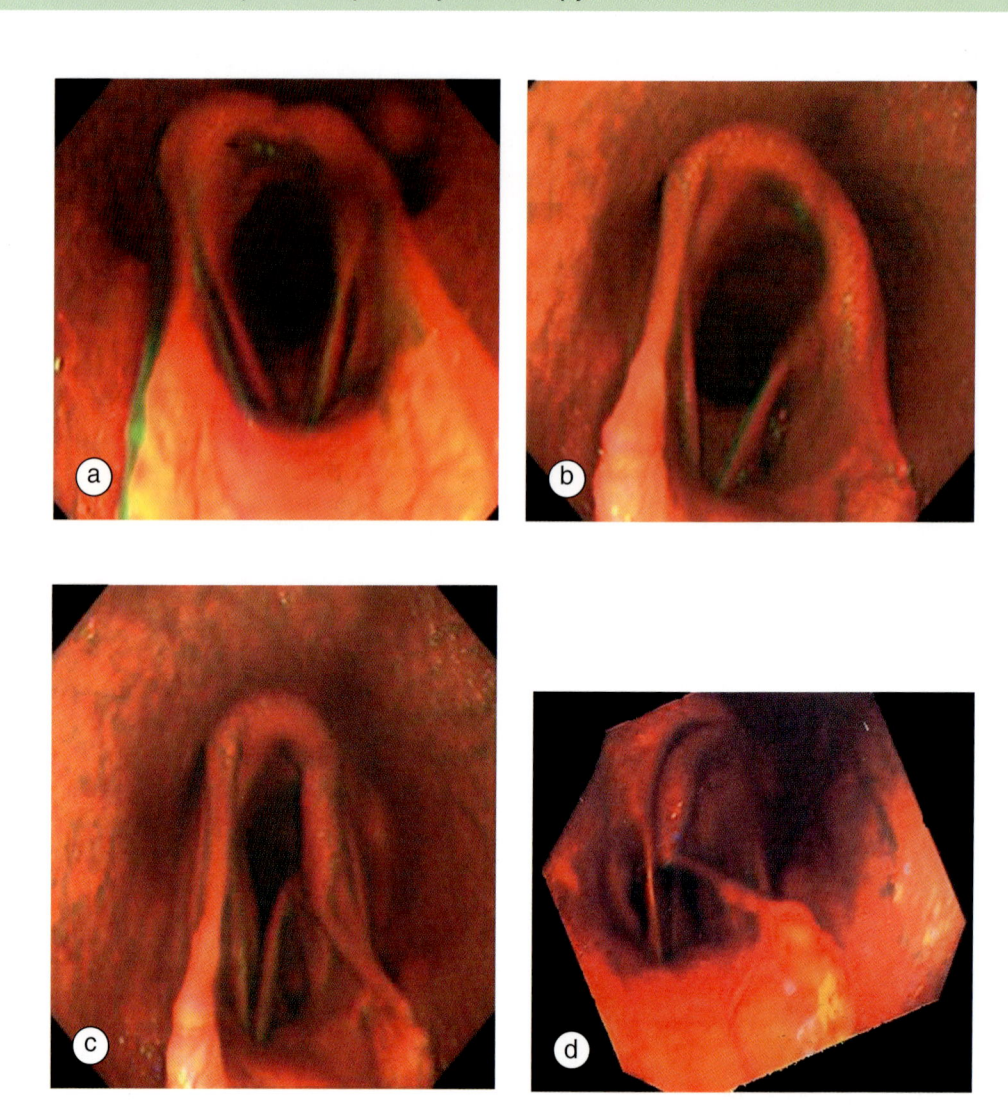

Fig. 8-6: Grade C laryngeal function during exercise.
a) At the beginning of exercise, the larynx is asymmetrical, but the left arytenoid maintains partial abduction.
b) As the horse begins to tire, the left arytenoid and vocal fold progressively collapse towards the midline during inspiration.
c) The left arytenoid begins to cross the midline.
d) The left arytenoid contacts the right arytenoid, completely obstructing the airway during inspiration.

exercise can collapse axially on inspiration and partially obstruct the airway (Fig. 8-5) without significant arytenoid collapse, and for these horses, vocalcordectomy or ventriculocordectomy may be an effective surgical treatment.

Chapter 8: **High-speed treadmill endoscopy**

Intermittent epiglottic entrapment

Entrapment of the epiglottic cartilage in the glossoepiglottic and aryepiglottic folds can usually be diagnosed in the resting horse, but the condition occasionally occurs only intermittently during exercise. In horses with epiglottic entrapment, pressure differentials generated within the nasopharynx force the free edge of the entrapping fold to be drawn ventrally towards the epiglottis during inspiration (Fig. 8-7a). During expiration, the entrapping membranes fill with air, ballooning outwards and often significantly obstructing airflow (Fig. 8-7b). Epiglottic entrapment, whether intermittent or persistent, frequently causes DDSP during exercise.

Treatment of epiglottic entrapment is discussed in Chapter 6.

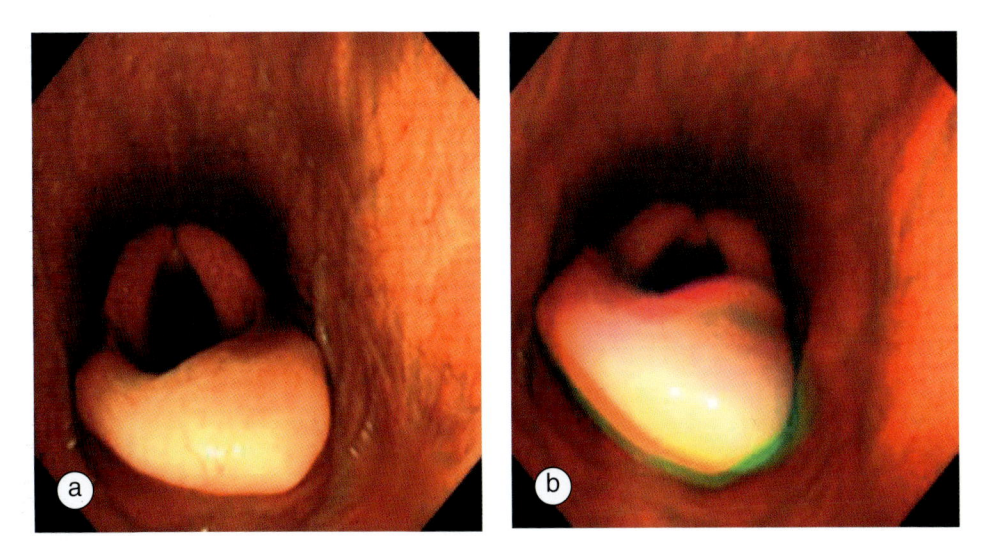

Fig. 8-7: Epiglottal entrapment.
a) During inspiration, the fold of mucosa entrapping the epiglottis is drawn ventrally towards the epiglottic cartilage.
b) During expiration, the mucosal fold is filled with air and balloons outwards, causing respiratory obstruction and a 'gurgling' noise.

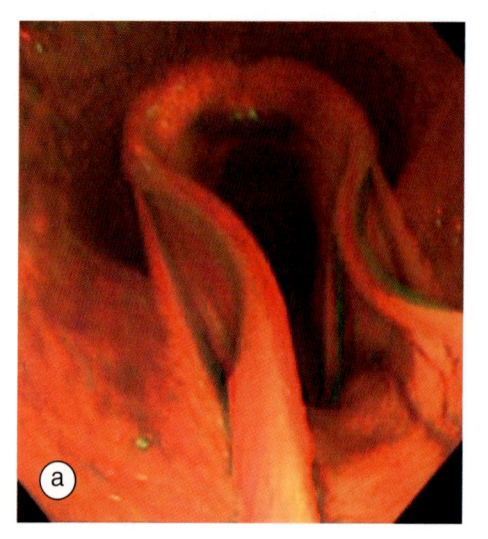

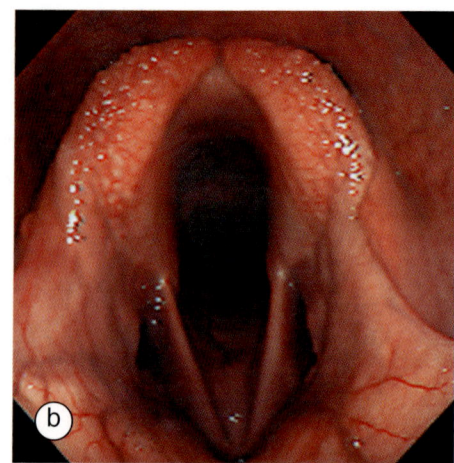

Fig. 8-8a: Severe bilateral axial deviation of the aryepiglottic folds. **b:** Aryepiglottic fold resection has been performed on the left side in this horse.

Table 8-2: Definition of mild, moderate and severe ADAF

Grade of ADAF	Definition	Obstruction of glottis (%)
Mild	Axial deviation of one or both aryepiglottic folds, with folds remaining abaxial to the vocal cords	<20
Moderate	Axial deviation of one or both aryepiglottic folds less than halfway between the vocal cord and midline	21–40
Severe	Collapse of one or both aryepiglottic folds more than halfway between the vocal cord and midline	41–63

Source: King DS, Tulleners EP, Martin BB, et al. 2001 Clinical experiences with axial deviation of the aryepiglottic folds in 52 racehorses. Veterinary Surgery 30:151–60

Axial deviation of the aryepiglottic folds (ADAF)

In horses with ADAF, the aryepiglottic fold (which extends between the corniculate process of the arytenoid cartilage and the lateral edge of the epiglottis) deviates axially on inspiration during strenuous exercise. Collapse of the arytenoid cartilage or dorsal billowing of the soft palate may remove tension from these folds, predisposing the horse to ADAF. Concurrent dynamic upper-airway disorders have been reported in 30–50% of horses with ADAF. This disorder is observed in many exercising horses to a mild, clinically insignificant degree (Figs 8-3b, 8-04) but occasionally can be characterized as moderate or severe (Figs 8-8a, 8-15) and can cause significant airway obstruction. The degree of deviation in some horses can progress from mild through to severe (Table 8-2), depending on the degree of fatigue.

Chapter 8: High-speed treadmill endoscopy

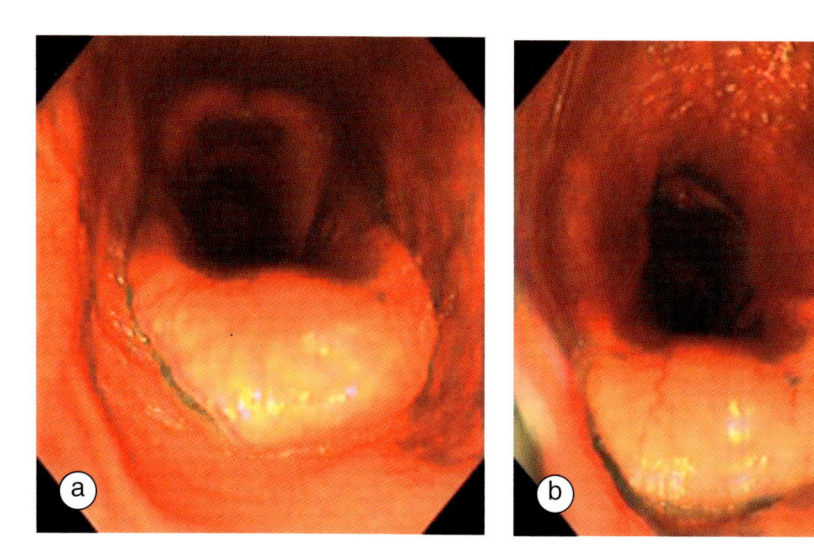

Fig. 8-9: Dynamic lateral nasopharyngeal collapse. During inspiration, **b)** the lateral walls of the nasopharynx are sucked axially, partially obscuring the rima glottidis.

Treatment of horses affected with ADAF usually involves resection of the offending portion of aryepiglottic fold (Fig. 8-8b), either via a laryngotomy incision or transendoscopically using laser surgery. This treatment has been reported to be successful in 75% of cases.

Nasopharyngeal collapse

The caudal two-thirds of the nasopharynx has no rigid support, and this area relies on neuromuscular function to resist collapse during inspiration. Dynamic nasopharyngeal collapse may therefore be related to neuromuscular dysfunction of the nasopharynx. The nasopharynx can collapse laterally (Fig. 8-9), circumferentially (Fig. 8-11) or dorso-ventrally

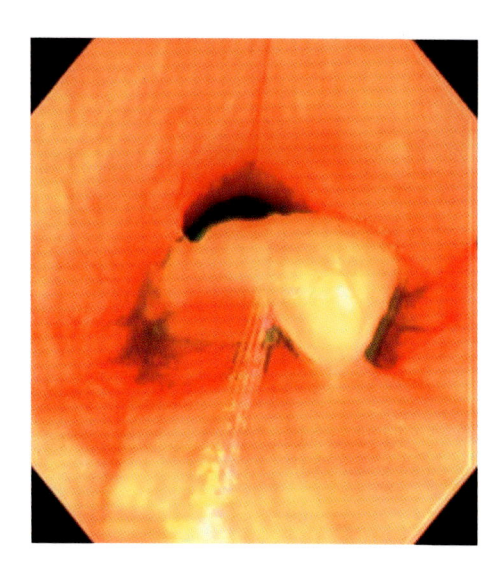

Fig. 8-10: Severe dynamic dorsal nasopharyngeal collapse. This photograph was taken during HSTE at inspiration. Note how the roof of the nasopharynx has collapsed ventrally to almost completely occlude the rima glottidis.

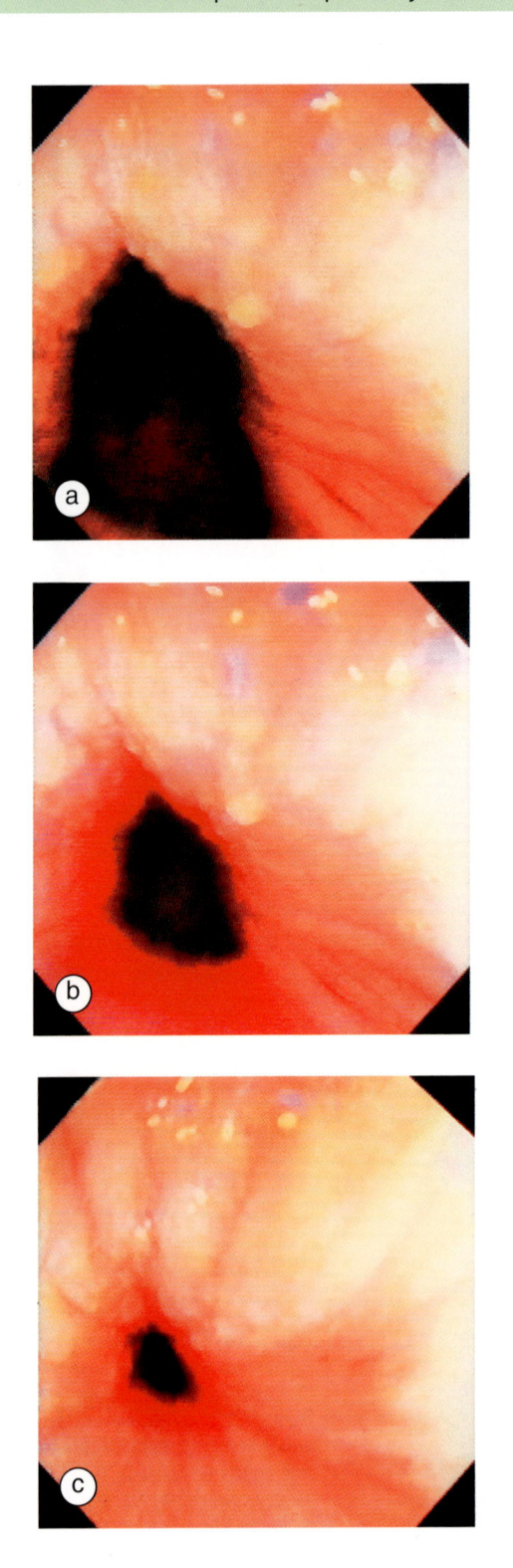

Fig. 8-11a–c: Circumferential nasopharyngeal collapse which occurred during HSTE during each inspiration, and which was associated with poor performance and considerable respiratory noise.

Chapter 8: **High-speed treadmill endoscopy**

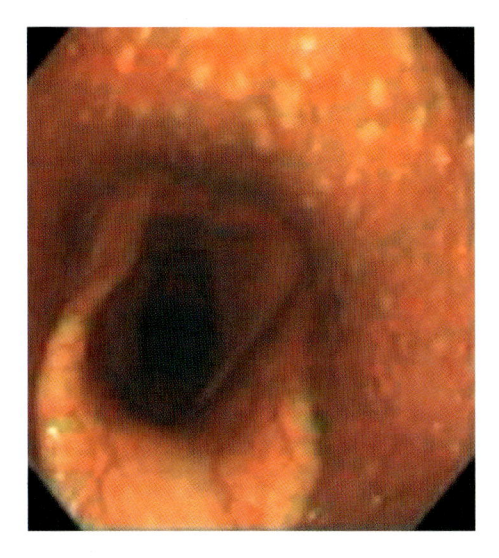

Fig. 8-12: Dynamic rostral displacement of the palatopharyngeal arch. This horse was normal on resting endoscopy, but during HSTE, the right palatopharyngeal arch (which is continuous with the aryepiglottic fold) has formed a 'cowl' over the right corniculate process. This horse was diagnosed with fourth branchial arch defect.

(Fig. 8-10). Collapse of the roof of the nasopharynx should be considered abnormal if it obstructs more than one-third of the rima glottidis. Lateral collapse of the nasopharynx that encroaches over the rima glottis should also be considered abnormal. In more severely affected horses, nasopharyngeal collapse is usually associated with loud abnormal respiratory noises. Some horses may develop the disorder only when the head and neck are flexed.

There is currently no effective treatment available for horses affected with nasopharyngeal collapse.

Fourth branchial arch defects (4-BAD, cricopharyngeal-laryngeal dysplasia)
The vast majority of horses with 4-BAD have abnormalities that can be detected during resting endoscopy, but in a small percentage of affected horses abnormalities may only become evident during HSTE. Abnormalities noted during HSTE include dynamic rostral displacement of the palatopharyngeal arch (Fig. 8-12), collapse of the right, left or both arytenoid cartilages and/or vocal folds (right-sided dysfunction is more common than left-sided or bilateral dysfunction in horses with 4-BAD), unilateral or bilateral ADAF and DDSP.

Epiglottic retroversion and axial collapse of the lateral margins of the epiglottis
Epiglottic retroversion is a rare disorder observed during HSTE, characterized by dorsal and caudal movement of the epiglottis (retroversion) into the rima glottidis during each inspiration. Although the epiglottis may become fully retroverted, the soft palate remains in its normal position at all times during the respiratory cycle in affected horses.
Axial collapse of the lateral margins of the epiglottis is diagnosed when the left or right edges of the epiglottis are observed to vibrate or displace axially during inspiration, often at the same time that an abnormal respiratory noise is created. It is sometimes associated with epiglottic hypoplasia or flaccidity, but the disorder may occur in horses with a normal epiglottic appearance at rest.

Bilateral arytenoid cartilage and vocal fold collapse

This disorder has been reported to be associated with head flexion in Norwegian Coldblooded Trotter racehorses, but it could occur in other breeds that are exercised with a similar head-carriage. When the head of an affected horse is flexed during HSTE, dynamic collapse of both vocal folds and reduced abduction of both arytenoid cartilages occurs (Fig. 8-13a). This abnormality may be due to inability of the arytenoid cartilages to abduct secondary to conformational changes in the throat region associated with head flexion and the use of particular tack in predisposed horses. Bilateral vocal fold collapse is occasionally noted in horses exercising with normal head carriage (Fig. 8-14b).

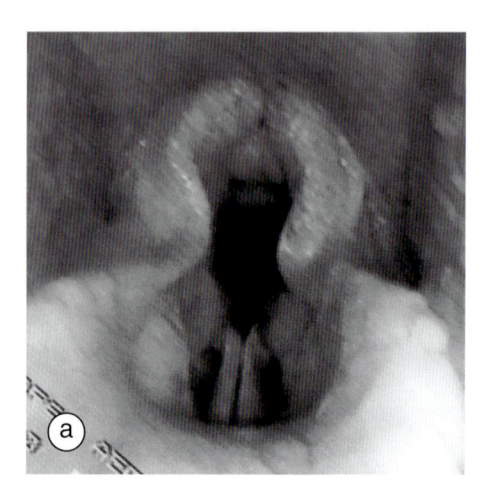

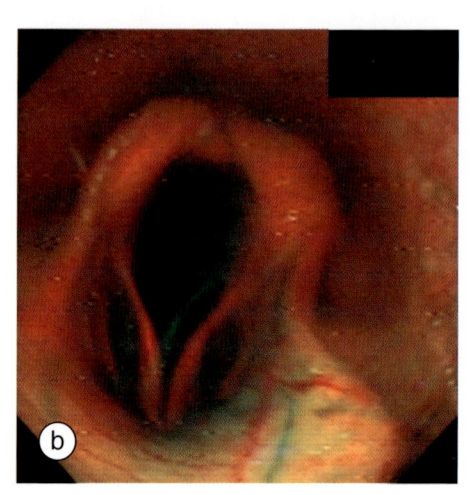

Fig. 8-13: Bilateral vocal fold/arytenoid collapse. **a):** HSTE photograph of a Norwegian Coldblood Trotter during exercise with induced neck flexion. There is bilateral loss of abduction of the arytenoid cartilages and bilateral axial collapse of the vocal folds and the aryepiglottic folds. The right lateral margin of the epiglottis is also mildly collapsed in an axial direction. Photograph courtesy E. Strand, Norwegian School of Veterinary Medicine. **b):** Bilateral vocal fold collapse with the arytenoids maintaining moderate abduction.

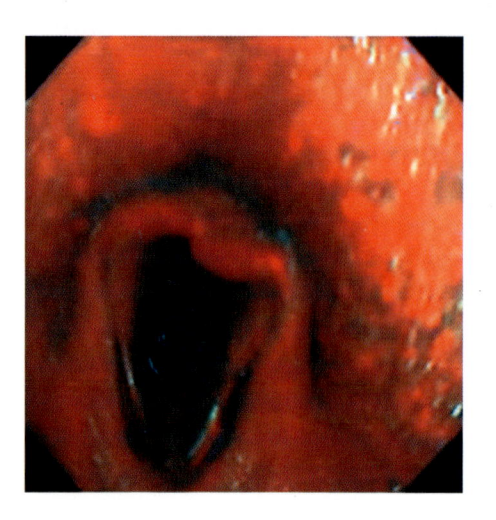

Fig. 8-14: Collapse of the apex of the corniculate process of the left arytenoid cartilage during HSTE. Note the ventral aspect of the corniculate process remains abducted. Photograph courtesy of P. Dixon.

Chapter 8: High-speed treadmill endoscopy

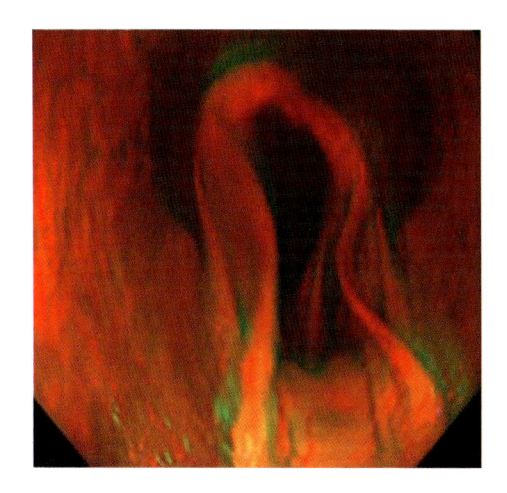

Fig. 8-15: Bilateral ADAF and grade B laryngeal function can be observed concurrently in this horse undergoing HSTE.

Collapse of the apex of the corniculate process of the left arytenoid cartilage (Fig. 8-14)

This disorder is an uncommon cause of upper airway dysfunction, but may affect the athletic potential of racehorses and other performance horses. The cause of the abnormality is unknown, but it is speculated that it may be an unusual manifestation of RLN. Affected horses exhibit progressive collapse of the apex of the corniculate process of the left arytenoid cartilage under the right arytenoid cartilage in the dorsal appostion of the two cartilages. This causes a partial obstruction at the dorsal aspect of the rima glottidis. The ventral aspect of the corniculate process remains abducted.

Multiple abnormalities (Figs 8-3, 8-13, 8-15)

Multiple abnormalities of the respiratory tract are commonly observed during HSTE in up to 50% of horses presented for investigation of abnormal respiratory noise or poor performance at exercise, and often, slow-motion playback of video/DVD footage is required to clearly identify all the abnormalities which occur.

FURTHER READING

Dart AJ, Dowling BA, Hodgson DR et al. 2001 Evaluation of high-speed treadmill videoendoscopy for diagnosis of upper respiratory tract dysfunction in horses. Australian Veterinary Journal 79:109–11

Hammer EJ, Tulleners EP, Parente EJ et al. 1998 Videoendoscopic assessment of dynamic laryngeal function during exercise in horses with grade III left laryngeal hemiparesis at rest: 26 cases (1992–1995). Journal of the American Veterinary Medical Association 211:399–403

Kannegieter NJ, Dore ML 1995 Endoscopy of the upper respiratory tract during treadmill exercise: a clinical study of 100 horses. Australian Veterinary Journal 72:101–7

Parente EJ, Martin BB 1995 Correlation between standing endoscopic examinations and those made during high-speed exercise in horses: 150 cases. American Journal of Veterinary Research 41:170–5

Tan RH, Dowling BA, Dart AJ 2005 High-speed treadmill videoendoscopic examination in the horse: the results of 291 clinical cases. Veterinary Journal 170:243–8

Chapter preview

Indications 119

Normal anatomy 120

Technique 124

    Trephination sites 125

Abnormalities 126

    Primary sinusitis 126

    Dental sinusitis 127

    Sinus cysts 128

    Progressive ethmoidal hematomas (PEH) 128

    Trauma 129

    Neoplasia 130

    Mycotic sinusitis 131

Further reading 132

Chapter 9: **Sinoscopy**

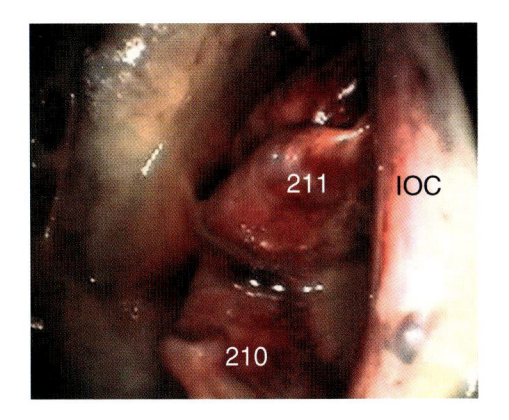

Fig. 9-6: Apices of cheek teeth 210 and 211 within the caudal maxillary sinus, lateral to the infra-orbital canal (IOC), viewed from a frontal sinus portal. Photograph courtesy of J. Perkins.

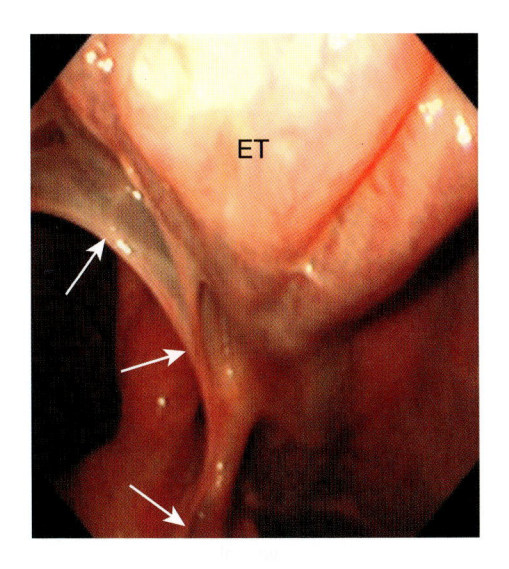

Fig. 9-7: Dorso-lateral aspect of the ethmoturbinates (ET) which are within the medial aspect of the conchofrontal sinus (viewed from an endoscopic portal in the frontal sinus). The fronto-maxillary aperture is marked by arrows.

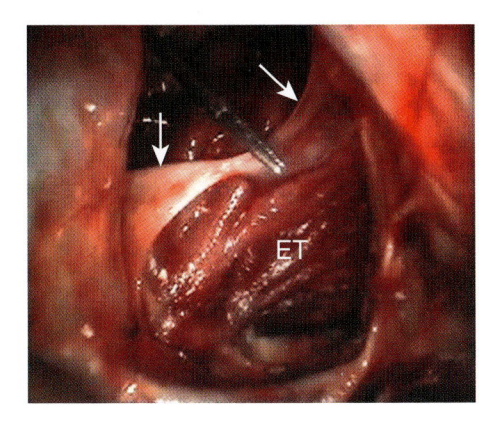

Fig. 9-8: Ventro-lateral aspect of the ethmoturbinates (ET) which are within the caudal maxillary sinus (viewed from endoscopic portal in the CMS). An instrument has been passed through a frontal sinus portal, and directed ventrally so that the tips are positioned just below the fronto-maxillary aperture (arrows). Photograph courtesy of J. Perkins.

The sphenopalatine sinuses consist of the sphenoidal and palatine sinuses which are situated at the caudo-medial aspect of the CMS, medial to the infra-orbital canal. The dorsal and lateral walls of the sphenoidal sinus are directly adjacent to cranial nerves II, III, IV, V and VI and also to major blood vessels. The ethmoidal sinuses lie within the larger of the ethmoturbinates and communicate with the CMS. This explains why some horses with sinusitis have grossly swollen and reddened ethmoturbinates, particularly ethmoturbinate no. 2, which can be observed endoscopically *per nasum* (Fig. 9-9).

Technique

Sinoscopy is a minimally invasive technique that can be performed on the sedated horse. If a small-diameter endoscope (e.g. 8 mm or less) is used, only a small trephine hole need

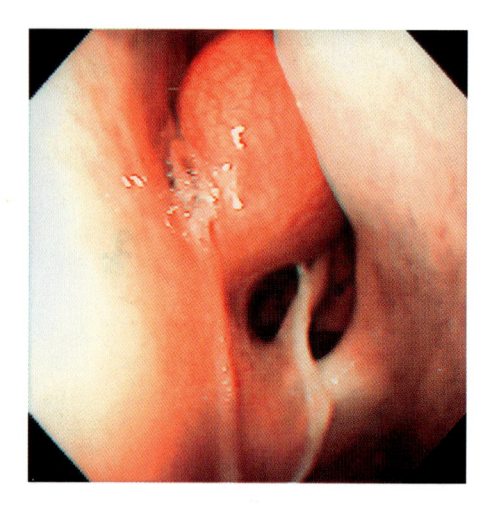

Fig. 9-9: Caudal aspect of the middle meatus of a horse with primary sinusitis, showing ethmoturbinate no. 2 which is very reddened. This is due to extension of infection from the caudal maxillary sinus to the ethmoidal sinuses. Mucopurulent discharge is emanating from around this ethmoturbinate.

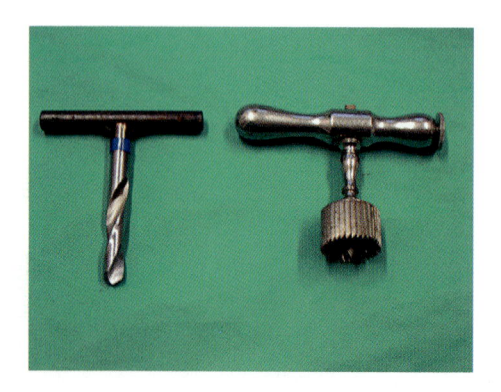

Fig. 9-10: Modified steel drill bit (left) and Galt trephine (right), either of which can be used for trephination of the sinuses.

Chapter 9: **Sinoscopy**

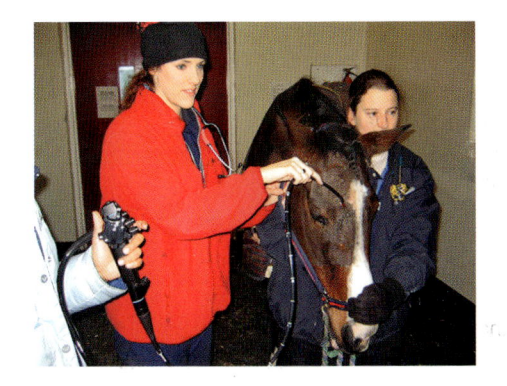

Fig. 9-11: Endoscope being introduced into a trephine hole in the frontal sinus. This horse has had a sinus flap surgery, and sinoscopy allows post-operative examination of the conchofrontal and caudal maxillary sinuses.

be made, and the endoscope can be more easily manipulated within the sinus. A small area of skin should be clipped and prepared for surgery, centered at the proposed trephination site, and local anesthetic is then injected subcutaneously. A 1.5 cm linear incision is made in the skin and underlying periosteum before the bone is trephined using a 1–1.5 cm diameter steel drill bit (Fig. 9-10), a Galt trephine (Fig. 9-10) or a large Steinmann pin. The endoscope is then introduced through this hole, into the sinus (Fig. 9-11). If the ventral parts of the sinuses are obscured by accumulation of purulent exudate, lavaging the sinuses before re-performing sinoscopy usually provides a clearer view.

Trephination sites

The frontal sinus portal is often the most useful, and allows examination of the frontal, dorsal conchal, caudal maxillary, ethmoidal and sphenopalatine sinuses. The site for this portal is positioned 0.5 cm caudal to a line drawn between the left and right medial canthi, and halfway between the midline and the ipsilateral medial canthus (Fig. 9-12). This is a particularly useful portal in young horses, whose cheek teeth occupy much of the maxillary sinus volume.

The maxillary sinuses of young horses are not often trephined for sinoscopy, because trephination of the maxillary bone risks damage to the reserve crowns and apices of the cheek teeth. Additionally, these long reserve crowns limit maneuverability of the endoscope inside the sinus and visualization of the intrasinus structures. The CMS portal (for sinoscopy of the CMS, sphenopalatine and conchofrontal sinuses) is positioned 2 cm rostral and 2 cm ventral to the medial canthus of the eye (Fig. 9-13). The RMS portal (for sinoscopy of the RMS and entrance to the VCS) is positioned halfway between the rostral aspect of the facial crest and the medial canthus of the eye, and 1 cm ventral to a line joining the infra-orbital foramen and the medial canthus (Fig. 9-13). The RMS portal in particular should not be used in horses less than 7 years old.

The RMS and VCS of most horses can also be examined endoscopically using a portal in the frontal sinus, if the ventral conchal bulla is removed. The bulla is relatively avascular and can be perforated using forceps introduced either through a separate instrument portal, or using the same portal as the endoscope (provided that the trephine hole is large enough to accommodate both; Fig. 9-5). After the dorsal part of the bulla is removed, a small

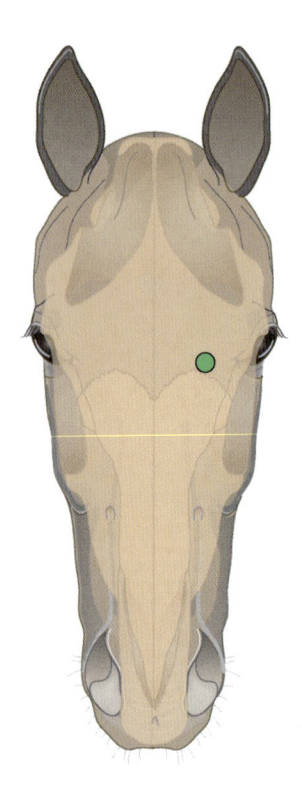

Fig. 9-12: Diagram of dorsal view of the horse's head, showing trephination site for the frontal sinus.

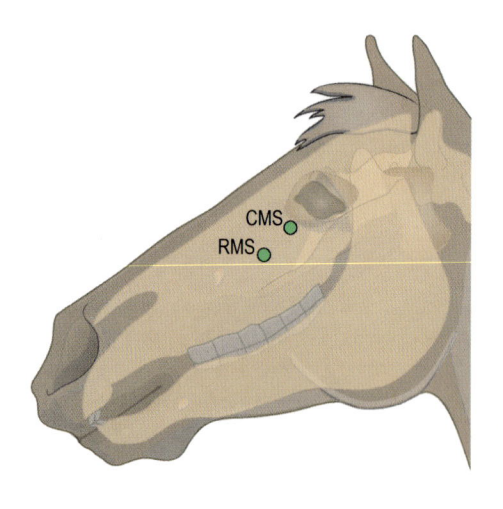

Fig. 9-13: Diagram of lateral view of the horse's head, showing trephination sites for the rostral (RMS) and caudal (CMS) maxillary sinuses.

endoscope can be passed medial to the infra-orbital canal to view the VCS or lateral to the infra-orbital canal to view the RMS.

Abnormalities

Primary sinusitis

Primary sinusitis is defined as inflammation of the sinuses in the absence of a detectable predisposing lesion. Primary sinusitis is thought to be caused initially by a viral respiratory infection, which results in a short-term, self-limiting, bilateral sinusitis, affecting all compartments. Failure of such cases to resolve due to impaired mucociliary clearance and reduced local mucosal defence mechanisms results in persistent sinusitis, which is often unilateral. Sinusitis is perpetuated by gross thickening of the sinus mucosa, which may obstruct the slit-like drainage ostium. If primary sinusitis is acute, mucosal thickening is mostly attributable to edema, but in more chronic cases, inflammation and fibroplasia additionally contribute to mucosal thickening. Horses with primary sinusitis commonly present with unilateral mucopurulent nasal discharge, which may be malodorous. Some affected horses may exhibit submandibular lymphadenopathy, facial swelling, epiphora and/or nasal obstruction.

Sinoscopy reveals liquid (Fig. 9-14) or inspissated (Fig. 9-15) purulent material in the sinuses, with no obvious predisposing cause. Treatment of acute cases of primary sinusitis consists of vigorous lavage using a catheter or length of plastic tubing implanted in the

Chapter 9: **Sinoscopy**

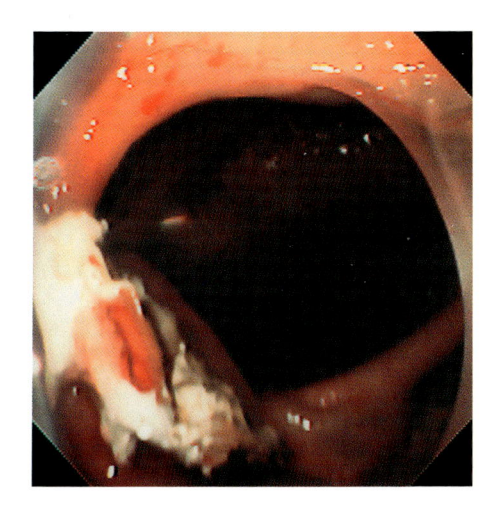

Fig. 9-20: Mycotic plaque at the rostral border of the fronto-maxillary ostium. Note the characteristic 'moldy cheese' appearance of this lesion. Mycotic infection was secondary to chronic primary sinusitis in this case.

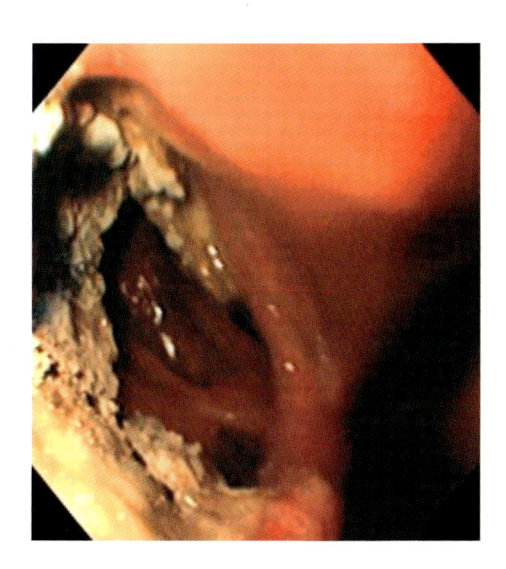

Fig. 9-21: Mycotic sinusitis. Caudal aspect of the right middle meatus (viewed with the scope passed *per nasum*) in a horse with primary mycotic infection of the sinuses. The fungal plaque has destroyed the medial wall of the ventral concha, creating a large sino-nasal communication.

Mycotic sinusitis

Mycotic sinusitis (Fig. 9-20) arises most commonly as an opportunistic infection after sinus surgery or secondary to some other sinus disorder, but occasionally it occurs with no other predisposing lesion present. Mycotic infections are often destructive, and occasionally cause large sino-nasal communications (Fig. 9-21). Clinical signs include malodorous unilateral nasal discharge and low-grade epistaxis. Treatment involves topical medication with an antifungal drug instilled into the sinuses via an indwelling catheter placed through a trephine hole.

FURTHER READING

Freeman DE 2003 Sinus disease. Veterinary Clinics of North America Equine Practice 19:209–43

Ruggles AJ, Ross MW, Freeman DE 1993 Endoscopic examination and treatment of paranasal sinus disease in 16 horses. Veterinary Surgery 22:508–14

Tremaine WH, Dixon PM 2001 A long term study of 277 cases of equine sinonasal disease. Part 1: Details of horses, historical, clinical and ancillary diagnostic findings. Equine Veterinary Journal 33:274–82

Tremaine WH, Dixon PM 2006 Sinoscopy. In: Equine Respiratory Medicine and Surgery. Eds: McGorum, Robinson, Schumacher, Dixon, Saunders

Index

NOTE: Page references in **bold** refer to photographs and illustrations.

Abscesses
  in the retropharyngeal lymph nodes, 57, **58**
  dental periapical, 23, **24,** 127
Adenocarcinoma, 22, 130
Aerophagia, 78
Artefacts, 11–12, **12**
Aryepiglottic folds, 67, **67, 116**
  see also Axial deviation of the aryepiglottic folds (ADAF)
Arytenoid cartilages, 67, **67, 68**
  chondritis, **74–7,** 76–8
  collapse, 105, 106, **116,** 116–17
  during exercise, **106, 109–10**
  mucosal defects, 76–7, **77**
  assymetry/asymchrony of, see Recurrent laryngeal neuropathy
Arytenoidectomy, 72, 75–6, **76**
Aspergillus fumigatus, **54,** 55–7
Auditory tubes, 49, **52,** 54, **54**
Axial deviation of the aryepiglottic folds (ADAF), 79, **79, 112,** 112–13, **117**

Biopsy and grasping forceps, 6, **6**
56
Bronchi
  normal anatomy,91, **92**
  tips for endoscopic examination, 91–4
Broncho-alveolar lavage, 12, 91–93, **94**

Carina, 89, 91, **91**
Catheters, **7,** 7–8
Caudal maxillary sinus (CMS), **120, 121–2, 122–3**
  Chemical restraint, 11
  see also Sedation
Choanal atresia, 27, **28**
Chondritis arytenoid, 74–6, **75–76**
Chondroids, 59–60, **59–61**
Chondroma, 99, **99**
Cleft palate, 41–2, **43**
Conchae, **15–18,** 15,19, **20**
Conchal sinuses, 120–4, **120–2**
Corniculate processes of arytenoid cartilages, 67 **67**
Cricoid cartilage, 67, **67**

Cricopharyngeal-laryngeal dysplasia see Fourth branchial arch defects
Cricopharyngeus muscles, 77
Cysts
  palatal, 46, **47**
  pharyngeal, 46, **48**
  sinus, 128, **129**
  subepiglottic, 83, **83**

Dental sinusitis, 127–8, **128**
Digastricus muscle, **51,** 53
Discharge from the sinus drainage angle, 24, **26, 119**
Disinfection of endoscopes, 5
Dorsal displacement of the soft palate (DDSP), 34
  intermittent, 38–40, **39,** 85, 105, **107,** 107–8
  persistent, 40, **41,** 83
Dysphagia, 36, **36,** 40, 55, 62, **73,** 76, 101, **101**

Empyema, guttural pouch, 57–8, **58–9**
Endoscopes, **3–4**
  accessories, 6–8, **6–7**
  maintenance of, 5–6
  selecting, 3–5
Epiglottis
  axial collapse of the lateral margins of the, 115, **116**
  cartilage, 67, **67**
  during exercise, **106**
  entrapment, 80–1, **80–2,** 83–5, 105, 111, **111**
  with DDSP, 39, **42**
  hypoplasia/flaccidity, 84–5, **85**
  retroversion, 105, 115
Epiglottitis, 84, **84**
Epistaxis, 12, 24, 55, **56,** 96, 129
Equipment, endoscopic, 3–8
Esophagus, **68**
Ethmoturbinates, 17, **18, 123,** 124, **124**
Eustachian tubes, 49, **52,** 54, **54**
Exercise-induced pulmonary haemorrhage (EIPH), 94–7, **96**
External carotid artery (ECA), **51,** 53, 62, **62**

Forceps, biopsy and grasping, 6, **6**
Foreign bodies

  nasal, 24, **27**
  nasopharyngeal, 44–46, **45–6**
  tracheal, 102
Fourth branchial arch defects (4-BAD), 77–9, **78–9,** 115, **115**
Fungal plaque, 55, **55,** 131, **131**

Galt trephine, **124,** 125
Glossoepiglottic mucosal fold, 33
Granuloma, 74, **75–76**
Guttural pouches, 49–64
  abnormalities/disorders of, 55–63, **55–63**
  empyema, 57–8, **58–9**
  guttural pouch mycosis (GPM), 36, **36,** 55–7, **54–56**
  lavage, 57, **60**
  normal anatomy, 49–53, **49–53**
  ostia, **32,** 34, **34,** 37, **38,** 57
  tips for endoscopic examination, **52–3,** 53–4
  tympany, **61,** 61–2

Heaves, 94, **95**
Hematoma, ethmoidal, **19,** 24, **25,** 128–9
Hemiplegia, laryngeal see Recurrent laryngeal neuropathy
High-speed treadmill endoscopy (HSTE), **105**
  abnormalities, 107–17
  normal anatomy, 106
Hobday procedure, 72, **73, 74**
Horner's syndrome, 55
Hyoepiglottic muscles, 33

Iatrogenic palate defects, **43,** 44
Infection of the rostral maxillary of cheek teeth, 23–24, **23**
Internal carotid artery (ICA), 50, **50**

Kerato-conjunctivitis sicca, 63
Kissing lesions, 74, **76**

Laryngoplasty, 72, **73,** 108
Larynx, 67–87
  abnormalities, 69–87
  during exercise, **106**
  hemiplegia, 69–73
  laryngeal function grading system, 70, 108–110

133

Index

Larynx, (cont'd)
  laryngeal nerve, left recurrent, 69
  normal anatomy, **67–8,** 67–9
  recurrent laryngeal neuropathy, 69–73, **71–72,** 108–11
  tips for endoscopic examination, 69
Lavage
  broncho-alveolar, 91, 93, 94
  guttural pouch, 57
Light sources, 5, **5**
Lingual tonsil, 33
Longus capitus muscle, rupture of, 63–4
Lymphosarcoma
  intrathoracic, **100**
  of the guttural pouches, 62
  of the nasal cavities, 22, **22**
  of the pharynx, 44, **44**
  sino-nasal, 130

Maintenance of endoscopes, 5–6
Maxillary
  artery (MA), **51,** 53, 62
  cheek teeth, **23,** 120, **123,** 127–8, **128**
  sinuses, 120–4,
  vein (MV), **51**
Meatuses, nasal 15, **15–19**
Melanomas, 62, **62**
Multiple dynamic abnormalities of the respiratory tract, 117
Mycosis
  guttural pouch, 36, **36,** 55–57, **54–56**
  mycotic sinusitis, 131, **131**
  nasal, 20, **21**
Myxoma, 99, 130

Nasal
  cavities
    abnormalities, 18–29
    normal anatomy, 15–17, **15–18**
    tips for endoscopic examination, 18
  mycosis, 20, **21**
  polyps, 20–1, **22**
  septum, 27, **28, 32**
Nasopharynx
  collapse, 37, **37,** 105, 113–15, **113–14**
  tips for endoscopic examination of, 34
Neoplasia
  guttural pouch, 62, **62**
  nasal cavity, 22–3, **22**
  pharyngeal, 44, **44–45**
  sinus, 130
  tracheal, 99, **99**

Nostril see Nasal cavities

Oropharynx, 31, **31,** 33, **33,** 34
Osteoma, 130
Osteosarcoma, 130

Palatal instability, **107,** 107–8
Palatoglossal arches, 33
Palatopharyngeal arch, rostral displacement of the, 11, 75, 78, **78,** 115, **115**
Paralysis, laryngeal, see Recurrent laryngeal neuropathy
Persistent dorsal displacement of the soft palate, 40, **41, 42, 43,** 83
Perspective artifacts, 11, **12**
Pharynx, 31–47
  abnormalities, 31–47, 35–47, **35–47**
  accumulation of respiratory secretions, 37, **38**
  normal anatomy, 31–4, **31–4**
  paralysis, **36,** 36–7, 55
  pharyngeal lymphoid hyperplasia (PLH), **35,** 35–6
  tips for endoscopic examination, 34
Plica salphingopharyngea, 54, **54**
Polyps
  nasal, 20–1, **22**
  tracheal, 99, **99**
Primary sinusitis, 126–7, **127**
Progressive ethmoidal hematomas (PEH) see Hematoma, ethmoidal
Pulmonary disease, 94, **95**

Rectus capitus muscle, rupture of, 63–4
Recurrent laryngeal neuropathy (RLN), 69–73, **71–4,** 108–10, **109–110**
Restraint of the horse, **11,** 11–12
  see also Sedation
Retropharyngeal lymph nodes, 37, **37,** 51, 54, **58,** 62
  abscess in, 57, **58**
Rhinitis sicca, 20
Rima glottidis, 67, **67,** 106
Roaring see Recurrent laryngeal neuropathy
Rostral displacement of the palatopharyngeal arch (RDPA), 11, **12,** 75, 78, **78, 115**
Rostral maxillary sinus (RMS), 120–121, **120**

Sedation, 11–12
  aerophagia, 78

broncho-alveolar lavage, 91
  effect on larynx, 69
Sino-nasal ostium, **18,** 26–7
Sinoscopy,
  abnormalities, 126–32
  indications, 119–20
  normal anatomy, 120–4
  technique, 124–6
Sinus, 120–132
  cyst, **20,** 128, **129**
  distension, 19
  drainage angle, discharges from, **26,** 26–8, **119**
  food material in, 128, **129**
  neoplasia, 130
  trauma, 129–30, **130**
  see also Sinoscopy
Sinusitis,
  dental, 127–8, **128**
  mycotic, 131, **131**
  primary, 126–7, **127**
Soft palate, 31, **31–3,**
  cleft palate 41–42, **43**
  iatrogenic defects 44, **43**
  see also Dorsal displacement of the soft palate (DDSP)
Squamous cell carcinomas, 22, 62, 99, 130
Steinmann pin, 125
Sterilization of endoscopes, 5–6
Storage of endoscopes, 6
Strangles, 57
Streptococcus equi var equi, 57
Stylohyoid bone, 49, **49, 50,** 55, 63, **63**
Stylopharyngeus muscle, 50, **50**
Subepiglottic
  cysts, 83, **83**
  ulceration, 86, **86**
Superficial temporal artery (STA), **51**

Teeth, maxillary cheek, 23, 120, **123,** 127–8, **128**
Temporal bone, 63
Temporohyoid osteopathy, 63, **63**
Thyroid cartilage, 67, **67,** 77
Tie back, see Laryngoplasty
Timing of examination, 12–13
Tongue, 33
Trachea
  abnormalities, 94–102
  collapse, 97–8, **97–8**
  normal anatomy, 89–91, **89–92**
  obstruction, 100, **100**
  tips for endoscopic examination, 91–4
  tracheal sump, 89, **90, 95**
  wash, 92–93, **93**

Index

Tracheostomy, 72
Tracheotomy tubes, tracheal obstruction following removal of, 100, **100**
Trauma
 sinus, 129–30, **130**
 tracheal, 101, **102**
Trephination sites, 125–6, **126**
Trephine hole, 119–20, 124–6, **125–6**
Tympany, guttural pouch, **61**, 61–2

Ulceration
 corneal, 63
 of arytenoid cartilage mucosa, 76–7, **77**
 subepiglottic, 86, **86**

Ventral conchal sinus (VCS), 121, **122**
Ventriculocordectomy, 72–73, **73–74**, 108
Videoendoscopes, 3–5, **4**

Vocal cordectomy *see* Ventriculocordectomy
Vocal folds, **67**, 68
 collapse, 71, 105, **109–10**, 116, **116**
 during exercise, **106**
Whitehouse approach, chondroid removal, 60, **61**
Wind test, 30
Wry nose, 27, **28**

135